Healing Touch

Healing Touch

A Resource for Health Care Professionals

DOROTHEA HOVER-KRAMER, EdD, RN
with contributing authors
Janet Mentgen, BSN, RN
Sharon Scandrett-Hibdon, PhD, RN

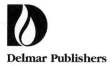

Delmar Publishers

I**T**P™ An International Thomson Publishing Company

Albany • Bonn • Boston • Cincinnati • Detroit • London
Madrid • Melbourne • Mexico City • New York • Pacific Grove
Paris • San Francisco • Singapore • Tokyo • Toronto • Washington

NOTICE TO THE READER

Cover Design: Spiral Design
Cover Illustration: Kirsten Soderlind

Delmar Staff
Publisher: David C. Gordon
Senior Acquisitions Editor: Bill Burgower
Assistant Editor: Debra M. Flis
Project Editor: Danya M. Plotsky
Production Coordinator: Barbara A. Bullock
Art and Design Coordinator: Mary E. Siener
Editorial Assistant: Chrisoula Baikos

Delmar Publishers' Online Services
To access Delmar on the World Wide Web, point your browser ↑
http://www.delmar.com/delmar.html
To access through Gopher: gopher://gopher.delmar.com
(Delmar Online is part of "thomson.com", an Internet site with information on more than 30 publishers of the International Thomson Publishing organization.)
For information on our products and services:
email: info@delmar.com
or call 800-347-7707

COPYRIGHT © 1996
By Delmar Publishers
a division of International Thomson Publishing Inc.

The ITP logo is a trademark under license.

Printed in the United States of America

For more information, contact:

Delmar Publishers
3 Columbia Circle, Box 15015
Albany, New York 12212-5015

International Thomson Publishing Europe
Berkshire House 168-173
High Holborn
London, WC1V 7AA
England

Thomas Nelson Australia
102 Dodds Street
South Melbourne, 3205
Victoria, Australia

Nelson Canada
1120 Birchmont Road
Scarborough, Ontario
Canada, M1K 5G4

International Thomson Editores
Campos Eliseos 385, Piso 7
Col Polanco
11560 Mexico D F Mexico

International Thomson Publishing GmbH
Konigswinterer Strasse 418
53227 Bonn
Germany

International Thomson Publishing Asia
221 Henderson Road
#05-10 Henderson Building
Singapore 0315

International Thomson Publishing—Japan
Hirakawacho Kyowa Building, 3F
2-2-1 Hirakawacho
Chiyoda-ku, Tokyo 102
Japan

6 7 8 9 10 XXX 01 00 99 98 97

Library of Congress Cataloging-in-Publication Data

Healing touch : a resource for health care professionals /
Dorothea Hover-Kramer.

p.   cm. — (Nurse as healer series)

Includes bibliographical references and index.

ISBN 0-8273-6275-7

1. Touch — Therapeutic use.   I. Title.

RZ999.H67   1996

615.8'52 — dc20

94–32097
CIP

INTRODUCTION TO NURSE AS HEALER SERIES

LYNN KEEGAN, PhD, RN, Series Editor

Associate Professor, School of Nursing,
University of Texas Health Science Center at San Antonio
San Antonio, Texas
and Director of BodyMind Systems, Temple, Texas

To nurse means to care for or to nurture with compassion. Most nurses begin their formal education with this ideal. Many nurses retain this orientation after graduation, and some manage their entire careers under this guiding principle of caring. Many of us, however, tend to forget this ideal in the hectic pace of our professional and personal lives. We may become discouraged and feel a sense of burnout.

Throughout the past decade I have spoken at hundreds of conferences with thousands of nurses. Their experience of frustration and failure is quite common. These nurses feel themselves spread as pawns across a health care system too large to control or understand. In part, this may be because they have forgotten their true roles as nurse-healers.

When individuals redirect their personal vision and empower themselves, an entire pattern may begin to change. And so it is now with the nursing profession. Most of us conceptualize nursing as much more than a vocation. We are greater than our individual roles as scientists, specialists, or care deliverers. We currently search for a name to put on our new conception of the empowered nurse. The recently introduced term *nurse-healer* aptly describes the qualities of an increasing number of clinicians, educators, administrators, and nurse practitioners. Today all nurses are awakening to the realization that they have the potential for healing.

It is my feeling that most nurses, when awakened and guided to develop their own healing potential, will function both as nurses and healers. Thus, the concept of nurse as healer is born. When nurses realize they have the ability to evoke others' healing, as well as care for them, a shift of consciousness begins to occur. As individual awareness and changes in skill building occur, a collective understanding of this new concept emerges. This knowledge, along with a shift in attitudes and new kinds of behavior, allows empowered nurses to renew themselves in an expanded role. The Nurse As Healer Series is born out of the belief that nurses are ready to embrace guidance that inspires them in their journeys of empowerment. Each book in the series may stand alone or be used in complementary fashion with other books. I hope and believe that information herein will strengthen you both personally and professionally, and provide you with the help and confidence to embark upon the path of nurse-healer.

Titles in the Nurse As Healer Series:

Healing Touch: A Resource for Health Care Professionals

Healing Life's Crises: A Guide for Nurses

The Nurse's Meditative Journal

Healing Nutrition

Healing the Dying

Awareness in Healing

Creative Imagery in Nursing

DEDICATION

*To all those who seek wholeness —
in their personal lives, in healing
relationships, and for our planet.*

CONTENTS

Chapter 3   Research Foundations, 27
Sharon Scandrett-Hibdon, PhD, RN

Part 2   THE HUMAN ENERGY FIELD, 43

P R E F A C E

Like many young persons of the early 1960s, I had a burning desire to do something useful amidst a time of increasing social awareness. Practicing music and writing papers for my first year of college seemed like remote and abstract activities, so I entered nursing despite my family's objections. Three years of a diploma program at Flower Hospital in Toledo, Ohio, gave me techniques and skills, but somehow the essence of caregiving was missing. I wondered when we would learn to heal with our hearts and hands as they did long ago. I kept asking the question and received puzzled looks from my instructors. The answer was to be much more complex and removed from my classes than I could imagine.

Gaining more nursing theory through bachelor's and master's programs at Boston University was stimulating, and I had some fine teachers. I began to realize that the healing work I hoped to find might be more subtle and less accessible than I thought. Perhaps answers would evolve from within if I kept asking and seeking. Perhaps we would just have to create healing environments in Western health care settings after learning from the East.

My family and I traveled to the Orient for 4 years and I practiced public health nursing in a variety of cultural settings in Singapore. The Chinese seemed generally embarrassed to admit they sometimes used herbs and acupuncture instead of Western medicine, and it was difficult to get much information from them. It seemed, at least then, they were determined to imitate our Western model, which was narrow in its focus.

Being educated in principles of prevention I sought out ways of preventing physical illness and began to find that emotional problems often appeared before the onset of physical disease. I thought if we could intervene at times of crisis, such as grief, childbirth, or family conflict, we might be able to prevent severe illness. This led to my exploring the mental health resources of Singapore, which were quite limited at the time, and to developing my skills as a counselor.

After returning to the States and reorganizing my family life, I studied psychology and received a doctorate in educational psychology from Nova University in 1978. Since that time I have been in private practice as a psychotherapist, first as director of a large multispecialty group in Tampa, Florida, for 12 years and now as a specialist in bereavement counseling and energy-based therapy in the San Diego, California, area.

In 1988 the American Holistic Nurses' Association (AHNA), of which I was a board member for 7 years, had the good fortune to connect with a nurse healer from Colorado named Janet Mentgen. Instead of talking or theorizing, she was practicing her own style of healing in a private office setting using a variety of ingenious techniques. She also had been teaching classes in her unique blend of skills for 10 years in the Denver area. It seemed here was the embodiment of what I had been seeking and I wanted to learn all the skills and find ways of teaching others. Through the AHNA we had the educational resources to develop Janet's material into sequenced, multilevel learning experiences that could be taught on weekends or in comprehensive training sessions. Through the national networks of the AHNA we had the organizational structure to develop the classes in various parts of the country. In the end of 1989 Janet and AHNA piloted two classes, one in Memphis, Tennessee, with Sharon Scandrett-Hibdon, and the other with me in Gainesville, Florida. The rest is history, as they say — in 5 short years the core faculty of Janet, Sharon, Myra Till-Tovey, and I have spearheaded the teaching of more than 8,000 nurses and health caregivers, with more than 250 classes held in the past year alone.

It remained to explore the underlying philosophy of this highly successful program and to present the concepts, techniques, and applications of Healing Touch in a comprehensive textbook that could serve as a reference to students and interested health caregivers alike. Again, the resources of AHNA gave us the linkage with Lynn Keegan, past president of AHNA and the series editor. She asked me if I would like to do the book. Would I! As an older, wiser counselor, I still hold the young nursing student who wanted to heal very close. I could not resist accepting the task on her behalf and for the many others like her.

However, this book is the work of many — the four core faculty members named previously who have held the light for the program over the past 5 years, the wise women of the AHNA leadership council, the many students and teachers who have each taught us in unique ways, the wisdom of the healing arche- type that is again taking form in a time when planetary healing is essential. To all of them, my heartfelt thanks for helping a dream vision to become a reality and for contributing their thoughts, ideas, and trust in the healing process.

This volume will provide the reader (and potential healer) with the basic concepts of Healing Touch as they are currently being taught in a comprehensive training program for health pro- fessionals. In our first part we look at the nature of healing and how it expands our vision of health care beyond the usual treatment of

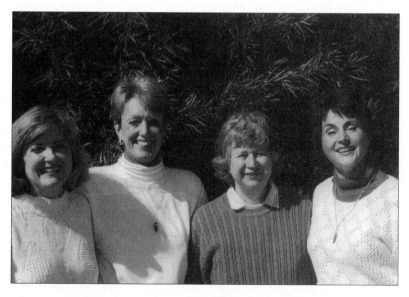

Healing Touch core faculty, left to right, Sharon Scandrett-Hibdon, Myra Till-Tovey, Janet Mentgen, Dorothea Hover-Kramer.

physical symptoms. The historical context for healing with energy-based approaches will be reviewed. We then give a brief overview of some of the most pertinent research.

In the first part, chapters 2 and 3 are written by Sharon Scandrett-Hibdon, PhD, RN, who is eminently qualified to bring her insights to these topics both as a member of the program advisory panel of the National Institute of Health (NIH) Office of Alternative Medicine and as an NIH funded researcher on endogenous healing. She is also the current president of the American Holistic Nurses' Association, a professor at the University of Tennessee in Memphis College of Nursing, and one of the four core faculty members for Healing Touch.

The second part addresses the specific knowledge and theory base that relates to the human energy field, its layers, and its energetic centers. In chapter 4 we discuss field theory and its practical implications for human caring. Chapter 5 describes the energy centers and their specific functions in the various dimensions of the field. In chapter 6, this information is integrated into an overview of sample patterns that may become evident in the field. The healer's assessment of the condition of the field leads to the application of the specific healing interventions that will be described in part 3.

The techniques described in the next four chapters are drawn from the beginning levels of the Healing Touch course and are presented in a way that makes them easy for you to use. Chapter 7 gives the basic tools for energy-related work in clinical settings with Therapeutic Touch as a home base. Chapter 8 explains full body techniques, and chapter 9 gives more specific and localized approaches. In chapter 10 we explore applications for specific client issues. Chapter 11 lists the actual components of a healing session and how one might develop a healing practice. It gives the identifiable steps of energy work and shows how healing is becoming accepted nationally through certification and other forms of recognition.

Chapters 7–11 are written by Janet Mentgen, BSN, RN. Janet helped to found, define, and administrate the Healing Touch program and has been an active nurse healer in the Denver area for more than 15 years. Currently, she is the program director of Colorado Center for Healing Touch, Inc., which coordinates all the

Healing Touch classes taught nationally and internationally by agreement with the American Holistic Nurses' Association.

One of the significant contributions of Healing Touch is that it integrates easily with other modalities the practitioner may already be using such as the many body-oriented therapies, traditional medical practice in hospital and clinical settings, and established practices of psychotherapy. In part 4 we will explore the bridges with medical settings, many of which are constantly developing as physicians and nurses utilize energy concepts as a complement to the work they are currently doing. Chapter 12 delineates this work via case examples to augment the existing research in clinical settings already described in chapter 3. In chapter 13, we learn about interfaces with several body-oriented therapies such as massage, polarity therapy, and Reiki. And in chapter 14, the numerous interrelationships with psychotherapy are described via case examples and practical applications.

Certainly, all healing work must begin with the practitioner's own healing. Although a perfect state of mental and physical health is an unrealistic expectation, a sense of direction or movement toward increasing wellness is essential. Because we as healers are role models through our relative wellness, we must begin by "walking our talk" — thinking, breathing, living, doing, and being — in a holistic way. This means that we respect the physical body and its needs, learn to release emotional tension, clear the mind of clutter, and connect with our spiritual essence on a daily basis.

In part 5, we offer applications of Healing Touch for the caregiver's own healing (chapter 15) and ways that the healer can increase self-awareness and personal development (chapter 16). Special thanks go to Myra Till-Tovey, BSN, RN, another core faculty member, for contributing her ideas to the latter chapter.

The conclusion summarizes our adventure of exploring the world of Healing Touch and opens to the many new questions that emerge as we apply the concepts. Enjoy our adventure!

F O R E W O R D

Late in the 1970s an explosion of interest in new approaches to health care emerged. In psychotherapy there was the advent of self-help programs, support groups, learning for personal growth, and self-awareness — the human potential movement as it came to be called. People no longer had to be mentally ill to want more out of life and to gain self-understanding. Getting help for a life crisis or transition became normal and acceptable. Better yet, people found that early intervention with physical or emotional needs prevented further deterioration or onset of chronic conditions.

In the 1980s this trend toward early intervention and increased self-care led to growing public interest in treatment modalities that went beyond usual medical approaches. In psychotherapy a variety of training programs in communication skills, interpersonal relationships, encounter groups, and the transpersonal dimension emerged. For care of the physical body a variety of alternatives gained public recognition, leading to mainstream acknowledgment of massage, chiropractic, acupuncture, and biofeedback. The formation of the American Holistic Nurses' Association (AHNA) and the American Holistic Medical Association (AHMA) in the early 1980s was inevitable on the crest of this wave.

In the 1990s the social and legal acceptance of these new modalities has become a major focus, with emphasis on health care reform, streamlining complex health care administration, and cost containment. New information about the complex interrelationship between the mind and the body has become available as well. Because of their effectiveness in preventing further disability, some unique approaches focusing on this interconnectedness have set a new standard of care. For example, Dr. Dean Ornish's program of stress management and imagery for persons diagnosed with cardiac symptoms is reimbursed by third party payers to assist in preventing the need for cardiac bypass surgery.

It is against this background of public interest in other ways of managing health care that approaches based on the human energy field and how it can be enhanced for healing can best be seen. Healing Touch, as presented in this book, is an example of such an approach. It is best understood as a complement or adjunct to other ways of treating the body/mind interconnection. Caregiving with Healing Touch involves internal preparation of the helping professional and specific techniques based on knowledge and skill. To further round out the picture, the history, research, and operating theoretical framework are presented with numerous applications and case examples. Beyond the basic understanding, however, no equipment is needed, allowing a welcome diversion from high-tech medical practice. The caregiver works with intuition, skill, a compassionate heart, and sensitive hands.

The energetic approaches, of which Healing Touch and Therapeutic Touch are best known in the health care field, have received increasing public interest and support. Many hospitals, notably in the Denver and Southern California areas, have policies that allow skilled practitioners of either modality to implement an energetic approach when appropriate. Health care consumers are requesting this work before and after surgery and in emergency and intensive care settings.

Let's explore now this fascinating resource for our clients and patients in this practical text and guide.

Dorothea Hover-Kramer,
Behavioral Health Consultants,
Poway, CA

1 | OVERVIEW, HISTORY, AND RESEARCH RELATED TO ENERGY-BASED HEALING

In the first part we will discuss concepts of healing via a heartwarming story, explore the historical information about energy-based healing work, and review the growing research literature about this work.

1 TOWARD AN UNDERSTANDING OF HEALING

Dorothea Hover-Kramer, EdD, RN and
Sharon Scandrett-Hibdon, PhD, RN

Within everything is the seed of perfect patterning.

Sharon Scandrett-Hibdon

Little Paul's Story

As I (Dorothea) outlined this chapter, wondering how best to begin, the telephone rang. "Hello, I'm Mary H. You probably don't remember me, but you helped my family for an hour three months ago and I shall never forget it." My mental computer quickly sorted for the British accent, the emotional tension in the voice, and, of course, I remembered. "Yes, you're little Paul's mother."

I felt my own emotions and tears as I recalled the hour that meant so much to Mary. A call came from a businessman who had read about Paul in the newspaper. The two-and-a-half-year-old boy desperately needed a bone marrow transplant for severe leukemia, but by the time the businessman had raised some money, the child was too ill for surgery. In desperation, the gentleman called me, having heard about Healing Touch through a friend. He wanted me to visit the family and fix everything. I attempted to explain about the complementary nature of energy-based work and that physical healing might not be the result of my visit. Undeterred, he insisted that I go to the family and share what I knew.

Although I agreed, I felt my resistance to the project. Why should I go, perhaps to help the child die? Then I remembered that often the various techniques of Healing Touch could be a resource when traditional medical practice, especially as we know it in the West, had reached the end of its capabilities. Steeled with this thought, I called the parents who expressed great eagerness to meet with me.

I got lost several times on my trip to a far part of the county, almost ran out of gas, and could not find a phone to tell them I was delayed. All of the obstacles seemed designed to test my resolve. When I finally arrived, I met Paul's older sister in the driveway and spent a few moments with her. Like many children in a family with severe illness, she seemed terribly alone in her fears and grief since the parents were totally absorbed with their little son.

A warm greeting from both parents assured me that I was not intruding. They were eager to learn about energy, and I shared some pictures of the human energy field. When I saw little Paul, I recognized the face of impending death. His skin was ash colored, his little eyes opened and rolled back in his head, and his breathing was labored and erratic. I recalled that energy-related therapy often facilitates easy transition to dimensions beyond this life. I felt there was a real possibility that Paul might pass on as I did Healing Touch with him.

Shoring up all the resources I could muster, I spoke with the parents about healing in other dimensions. If the physical could not improve, we might see a balancing in the emotions, increased mental clarity, or direct connecting with the spiritual/intuitive dimensions. They understood my meaning and asked me to help in any way I could. "You see, the doctors gave up on Paul over a week ago. We feel abandoned since they said there is nothing further they could do. We are obviously in need and Paul is still alive. Please stay with us awhile."

My heart reached out to them and their dilemma. As the father and mother took turns holding the frail body, I began smoothing the child's energy field. Whenever I came closer than two feet, Paul would whine a little and brush me away, so I knew the boundaries of his energetic field and continued the motion at a distance. I followed with some other Healing Touch techniques and a gentle transfer of energy above the heart center. I also taught the parents how to balance their own heart centers to increase relaxation and immune system functioning.

Fully expecting Paul to sleep or pass on, I was amazed when he clearly said, "I want milk" after about twenty minutes. His eyes became more alert, and, after finishing his milk, he wanted to go for a bike ride. When I left, Paul was sitting upright on his own in his little chair waiting to go for a ride with his dad. I looked into his eyes and saw the clear gaze of eternity looking back at me.

The next day was Good Friday, and I dreamed that Paul had left his physical body. The Monday after Easter his father called to tell me that Paul had, indeed, died on Good Friday but not until he had played with the family for three hours and everyone, even relatives, had been able to say farewell. "That Thursday afternoon was the greatest gift we could ever have received," his father said. "It was just like old times: we played and laughed and ate and slept soundly that night. The next morning both my wife and I told Paul that we would understand if he needed to go on. We were ready to release him, and in twelve hours he was gone."

THE IMPACT OF ENERGY-BASED WORK

What amazed me as a bereavement therapist was the healing that seemed to have occurred in the family. It is always difficult to release a precious child, but to do it in consciousness and with such clarity is remarkable. There truly seemed to be exquisite timing in the events just as they had unfolded. My presence somehow facilitated growth for this family in ways that might have taken months of more traditional grief therapy. The brief shift in little Paul's condition, physically and mentally, allowed a new dimension of awareness to emerge. The spiritual opening to Higher Power, the bigger picture as we might say, permitted the parents to gain a new perspective.

I continue to be amazed by and respectful of energy-based work. I know I did not myself bring these changes about, but I was privileged to be there as a facilitator. Mary repeatedly affirmed, "You gave us three hours with Paul we would never have had otherwise. We and our whole family are eternally grateful."

That Thursday afternoon was an incredible gift for me as well. I recognized that all parts of my training as a nurse, bereavement counselor, student of transpersonal psychology, and Healing Touch practitioner were needed in my interaction with the family. I felt blessed to have had a brief moment with this family in their time of need and to have helped them. I, too, felt that I was somehow made whole by the experience.

DEFINITIONS OF HEALING

Little Paul's story describes a form of emotional and intuitive healing at the time of a physical death. This seems like a paradox to most of us with analytical training and leads us to ask more extensively about the nature of healing as a creative process toward wholeness.

The word *heal* is derived from the Old English *haelen*, the Germanic *heilen*, and the Greek stem *holos*. *Merriam-Webster's Collegiate Dictionary* gives "to make sound or whole" as the primary definition, whereas "to cause an undesirable condition to be overcome or mended" is secondary. Even the more commonly used word, *cure*, is defined as "something which corrects, heals, or alleviates a harmful or troublesome situation." It is derived from *cura*, the Latin word for care of souls. So we see that ideas of restoration, bringing to wholeness, and attention to the spiritual dimension have been part of the vocabulary of healing for a long time.

More recent interpretations, especially in the West, hold that someone who is ill or who has physical symptoms is in need of a cure to return to the more symptom-free state that we call health. Inherent in the concept of healing is a wider, more integrative interpretation of our human reality; namely, we are physical beings with a material body, but we are also emotional beings with feelings that influence the physical, mental, idea-generating beings with thought patterns that influence our bodies and emotions, and, most importantly, spiritual beings having our human experience in a physical body, ultimately connected to the Creative Source.

One way of understanding healing is to consider it a multidimensional process toward ever-increasing levels of wellness in every part of our reality, even when there is an ongoing, or chronic, physical problem. In other words, things are not just black or white we are not just sick or well but are on a continuous spiral of evolution toward well-being and wholeness.

Another way to approach our exploration is by seeing all of life as a continuous flow. The flow can be harmonious or torturous. Healing implies movement from a disturbed or complex flow to a more harmonious one. This harmony encompasses the internal states within our organism as well as our relationships with the rest of the environment, our family, our community, and the world.

The process of healing is conceptualized as an integral part of a functioning whole organic process. Martha Rogers, a well-known nursing theorist, views healing patterns as movement of energy toward harmony of the human and environmental fields (Rawnsley, 1985). Another nursing leader, Janet Quinn (1993), describes harmony as finding right relationships between persons and their environment. Both definitions broaden our sense of healing to a larger context of harmonious interaction with our surroundings.

DEFINITIONS OF ILLNESS

Illness, in contrast, is an imbalance or disruption within the organism. It is a dysfunctional adaptation made in response to the environment. The presence of pain or discomfort, then, is a feedback signal that allows us to learn more about ourselves, our physical and emotional makeup, and our surroundings.

Symptom removal is the approach of most current health care practices to the dysfunctional pattern or *dis-ease*. The giving of medication to remove pain and surgical removal of a dysfunctional body part are major physical approaches to illness. These approaches do not provide healing in the broader sense that we are using. In the story of little Paul, physicians ended their attentions when it became evident that Paul's body could not improve. It is clear, however, that much more help of a different, creative nature could be offered.

Of course, symptom-removal thinking extends well beyond our health care model to societal interventions that focus on eradication of symptoms. An example of this type of thinking is the ongoing attempt to create crime-free neighborhoods through the elimination of its symptoms by locking up all lawbreakers. We can see that eradicating symptoms is a temporary measure at best. It serves as a cure that does not provide the deep transformation needed for genuine healing.

Healing is by its very nature restorative and prevents further disruptive patterns. Transformative healing allows us to move to a higher level of functioning, which creates harmonious connections with all of our environment.

DOCUMENTATION OF HEALING

Healing has been a practice of humanity for thousands of years. Whereas most medical writings are restricted to concepts of wound healing, many writings on the philosophy of healing are found in anthropological and philosophical literature (Henderson & Primeaux, 1981; Rush, 1981; Scott, 1974). However, documentation of healing as a transformative process encompassing body, mind, and spirit is sparse.

In a psychiatric journal article, Dr. A. Comfort (1978) describes healing as "reordering of the self and the acceptance of responsibility for health." Positive changes in our thoughts, emotions, or consciousness can bring about physiological alterations and thus are also considered to be healing (Meek, 1977). Rawnsley (1985), a nurse, defines healing as energy patterning, as motion that is facilitated toward harmony of human and environmental fields. Another definition is obtaining harmony and balance in relationship with one's deity (Rush, 1981). Rene Dubos (1980) identifies two types of healing — first, a reactive healing process that returns the individual to an earlier condition of homeostasis and second, a responsive healing process that is creative and evolutionary.

This brief review suggests there is a growing interest in healing, its mechanisms and interventions. Further exploration of the history of healing and its implications follows in the next chapter to give us a better understanding of what is actually involved in healing. Because healing takes place within the individual, we learn about it most directly from the clients, the patients. We can understand the internal, endogenous nature of healing by observing the progression toward improved levels of functioning.

SUMMARY

Healing is movement toward health, harmony, and wholeness. One way of conceptualizing healing is to think of it as repatterning of energy to a more harmonious vibrational frequency. To put it another way, right relationship with ourselves and others occurs as healing unfolds.

This book focuses mainly upon Healing Touch, the healing interventions that address repatterning and alignment to higher levels of functioning through working with the human energy field. These interventions are natural and assist the innate healing process. They promote repatterning of energy within the whole being, allowing balance, harmony, and right relationship to emerge. Human caring and touch assist the individual to relax, which allows for expansion and balance of the energy field. The healer uses energy from the Universal Energy Field to enhance the energetic field of the client, increasing opportunity for the healing to occur. A Healing Touch intervention often creates pathways from deep within that provide opportunity for the client to move to increasing health and wholeness.

This movement involves the whole person — the physical, emotional, mental, and spiritual — in energy changes that we will explore in the different parts of this book. Healing comes from within the individual, not from the healer. Yet, the healer may also be deeply touched and experience energetic and health changes simultaneously.

References

Comfort, A. (1978). On healing Americans. *Journal of Operational Psychiatry, 9:1:6*, 25–36.

Dubos, R. (1980). Health and creative adaptation. In Flynn (Ed.), *The healing continuum*. Bowie, MD: Robert J. Brady Company.

Henderson, G., & Primeaux, M. (1981). Religious beliefs and healing. *Transcultural health care*. Menlo Park, CA: Addison-Wesley Publishing Company.

Meek, G. W. (1977). *Healers and the healing process*. Wheaton, IL: The Theosophical Publishing House.

Quinn, J., & Strelkauskas, A. (1993). Psychoimmunologic effects of Therapeutic Touch on practitioners and recently bereaved recipients: A pilot study. *Advances of Nursing Science, 15*(4), 13–26.

Rawnsley, M. M. (1985). HEALTH: A Rogerian perspective. *Journal of Holistic Nursing, 3*(1), 25–29.

Rush, J. E. (1981). *Towards a general theory of healing*. Washington, DC: University Press of America.

Scott, C. S. (1974). Health and healing practices among five ethnic groups in Miami, Florida. *Public Health Reports, 89*, 524–532.

THE HISTORY OF ENERGY-ORIENTED HEALING

2

Sharon Scandrett-Hibdon, PhD, RN

---

*Evolution builds complexity and knowing. As we
record our history may we avoid re-creating mistakes.*

Sharon Scandrett-Hibdon

INTRODUCTION

Healing with energy and working with energetic principles is one
of the oldest forms of health care known to humankind. The ear-
liest Eastern evidence of energetic healing is in the *Huang Ti Ching
Su Wen* of 2,500–5,000 years ago (Veth, 1949). Similarly, pictures
of energy healing from the Egyptian Third Dynasty demonstrate
energetic conceptualization (Pavek, 1993). Ideas of energy centers
related to the human body and of an energetic envelope extending beyond the physical, known as the ka, were well known more
than 5,000 years ago in ancient Egypt (Hover-Kramer, 1993).
Imhotep, the builder of the famous step pyramid, was known to
be a talented healer. He became the formative idea for the Greek
deity of medicine, Aesculapius, thousands of years later.

EARLY ENERGETIC BELIEFS

In classical Greece, Hippocrates acknowledged the *biofield*,
another word for energy, as a force flow from many people's
hands. Pythagoras, in the Greece of 500 B.C., referred to vital

energy perceived as a luminous body that could produce cures. In medieval Europe, Paracelsus referred to vital force and matter, calling the energy *illiaster* (Brennan, 1993, p. 16). Other terms for energy or biofield are given in table 2.1 suggesting the universality of energy concepts.

Shamanic Contributions

Early shamanic work did not specify the biofield but utilized massage and magical rituals around the patient to restore proper rela-

Energetic Name	Cultural Source
Animal Magnetism	Mesmer
Ankh	Ancient Egypt
Arunquiltha	Aborigine (Australia)
Bioenergy	US/England
Biomagnetism	US/England
Gana	South America
Ki	Japan
Life Force	General Usage
Mana	Polynesia
Manitou	Algonquian
M'gbe	Hiru Pygmy
Mulungu	Ghana
Mumia	Paracelsus
Ntoro	Ashanti
Ntu	Bantu
Oki	Huron
Orenda	Iroquois
Pneuma	Ancient Greece
Prana	India
Qi (Ch'i)	China
Sila	Inuit
Subtle Energy	US/England
Tane	Hawaii
Ton	Dakota
Wakan	Lakota

From unpublished NIH-OAM Report: *Manual Healing Methods: Physical and Biofield* by Richard Pavek, 1994. Reprinted by permission.

TABLE 2.1 Some Equivalent Terms for Biofield

tionships. These relationships dealt especially with aligning the energies between humans, nature, and the spiritual world (Rush, 1981).

Eastern Contributions

In Far Eastern cultures, movement of life energy along meridians was a central concept in healing systems. Acupuncture and pressure points were stimulated to balance opposing energies, referred to as *yin* and *yang*. Blocked energy was believed to produce illness. *Sinarteriology* was the science of channeling *ch'i*, or life force energy, through the energetic flows in the body and stimulating the patient's energy in relation to the energy of the universe (Keegan, 1988). In ancient India, the *chakras*, which are human energy vortices invisible to the naked eye, were identified in the Ayurvedic approach of medicine. Activation of the chakras was used in self-healing, and the energy centers were balanced through the practice of yoga (Keegan, 1988). The extensive literature on the chakras and our current understandings of them will be addressed in chapter 5.

ENERGETIC CONCEPTS IN RELIGIOUS AND SPIRITUAL THOUGHT

In the Christian Era, healers were considered to be holy or mystical. There are 41 references in the New Testament to Christ's ability to heal, even as patients touched his garment. When Pope Alexander III issued an edict in the twelfth century to stop the healing mission of the clergy, some healers continued, such as St. Patrick of Ireland who healed the blind and St. Bernard of France who healed blindness, muteness, lameness, and deafness (Krieger, 1987). Healing circles and services are seen in today's religious practices as well. The spiritual infusion of healing has been an important influence since Christian times, allowing us to sense the "presence of God in all matter" and to see "the image of Christ in every man" (Keegan, 1988, p. 62).

Prominent Healers

Prominent healers, known throughout time, were special individuals honored in their society. Often they had rich internal lives.

Evidence of this exists in primitive cultures (Elkin, 1978; Katz, 1982; Landy, 1977). Krieger (1987) described how the interaction of one's cultural worldview and life experience colors understanding of the healing act. For example, some believe the source of healing is their own creation, others claim God creates the energy, and others believe the energy comes from one's ancestors.

Some prominent healers from early times include Thrita in Russia, identified from cuneiform tablets; Dhen Wantori from India; and the Greek Galen, who was physician to the Roman emperor Marcus Aurelius. Royalty were assumed to have healing power, and in England and France, royal cures of goiter and throat conditions were reported. The Roman emperor Hadrian cured dropsy, and the emperor Vespasian healed neurological disorders, lameness, and blindness. Valentino Greatrakes, a seventeenth century Irish landowner and magistrate, treated the ill without touching the body. He worked mostly with paralysis, deafness, swellings of tumors, and arthritis. In 1666 he toured London offering healings (Krieger, 1987).

Recent well-known healers include a Mexican from the nineteenth century, who was apotheosized by the Roman Catholic Church to religious folk sainthood, and more recently Olga Worrall, Oscar Estebany, Dolores Krieger, Dora Kunz, Rosalyn Bruyere, Barbara Brennan, and Janet Mentgen. Many of these healers' students also have great healing power and will be named in history.

THE USE OF ELECTROMAGNETICS

There is also a biomedical and electromagnetic history in physics that supports energetic healing. In the nineteenth century, Mesmer, Liebnitz, and Reichenbach cited aspects of electromagnetic field phenomena such as the attraction and repulsion of magnets to each other (Brennan, 1993). In the early twentieth century, Kilner observed the human aura using colored screens and filters to see three layers. He also correlated auric configurations and disease states. Emanations from the auric field were detected by George de la Warr in the 1940s through radionic instruments. These instruments were used for diagnosis and distance healing. Wilhelm Reich in 1930 to 1950 developed a model of psychotherapy utilizing the human energy field. Later, Burr and Northrup observed the life field that demonstrates organization of the human energy field and developed the concept of circadian rhythms. They found that measurements of the energy field of seeds correlated with the strength or weakness of plants and that weakness of the life field of animals predated disease. This work was furthered by Ravitz in the 1950s, who observed thought fields that interfered with the life field to produce psychosomatic symptoms (all the preceding cited in Brennan, 1993, pp. 16–17).

In the 1960s, Bernard Grad attempted to demonstrate separation of energy transfer from psychic ability. It was his concept that healing went beyond belief and charisma. He studied three groups of people including healers, a control group, and depressed persons. He then examined their effects on plant growth. Grad was attempting to demonstrate that there is an actual energetic effect that occurs in healing, which is unrelated to charisma or psychic ability. To do this, he used seedlings that were damaged in salt water and had healers hold the water that was later used on the plants. These plants grew stronger and more plentiful than the control seedlings. He further demonstrated that depressed patients produced negative effects on the growth of plants (Grad, 1979).

The Japanese researcher Motoyama developed a machine that electrically measured the acupuncture meridians for diagnosis in acupuncture treatment. Meridians are the energy flow lines coursing through the physical body that are studied and manipulated in acupuncture treatment. His 1981 study of energy, called *ki* in Japanese, found that meridians seem to exist in the dermal layer of connective tissue and have a direction of flow that can be detected. *Yin* energy flows upward; *yang* energy moves downward. The *ki* energy flows more slowly than galvanic skin response and nervous conduction. The *ki* also gathers in an affected meridian or organ, undergoes a transduction into a physiochemical energy or action potential, and can be detected by some individuals through sensory nerves. There seems to be a high center in the brain that controls the *ki* energy movement, according to Motoyama. The energy is also controlled by general physiochemical laws. When energy is flowing in different directions than it is supposed to, it is slowed down. Reverse flows have a lower amount of *ki* energy, whereas an excess of *ki* flows more rapidly (Motoyama, 1981, p. 73).

Uses of Electricity in Healing

Another application of energetic concepts in medicine is the use of electricity to promote healing and to reduce pain. In the past two decades the orthopedist Robert Becker has measured direct current control systems in relation to the human body in health and disease. His most revolutionary work was stimulating the body's tissue to regenerate bone (Brennan, 1993; Gerber, 1988). He also stimulated regeneration of frog's limbs, which normally does not occur, by reversing the polarity of the electrical charge. Dr. Becker also demonstrated repair of compound fractures of horses by implanting bone electrodes in the cast, which pulsed currents across fracture sites. Other specialists (Stavish & Horwitz, 1987; Taubes, 1986) used electric currents to reduce tumor size and to clear cancers in difficult places to treat such as in the lung.

Therapy with the use of magnets has also been found helpful in rheumatoid and degenerative arthritis (Rose, 1987). Magnets were placed on either side of joints for one or two treatments per day for 10 to 15 sessions on nearly 200 rheumatoid and degenerative arthritic patients. Results showed improvement in 73% of the rheumatoid patients and in 67% of the degenerative joint patients.

Norman Shealey, MD (1979) developed the Dorsal Column Stimulator, which utilized a weak electric current to alleviate intractable pain syndromes. This stimulator was surgically placed in the patient's lower spine to close the pain gate. Less intrusive pain gate closers have been developed since, such as the transcutaneous nerve stimulators that also use electricity to diminish pain sensation (Gerber, 1988).

ENERGY UTILIZATION IN MEDICINE

There are many other forms of energy utilization in medicine. Madame Curie's discovery of radium led to the widespread use of X rays, which are also energetic phenomena (Gerber, 1988). CAT scans and MRI techniques track hydrogen atoms in the body, and images of their energetic emanations are interpreted by computers to yield a picture of the body's functioning. Zimmerman used the ultrasensitive SQUID (superconducting quantum interference device) to detect weak but significant increases in the magnetic field emanations of healers' hands during healing. He also measured brain waves, finding a right to left brain synchronization in the alpha, or meditative, state. He conjectures that grounding techniques, which healers use to focus themselves, are a connecting into the earth's magnetic field to develop a synchronization of the healers' brain waves with the frequency of the earth's electromagnetic envelope (Brennan, 1993, p. 17).

Kirlian Photography

Kirlian photography, a special photographic process that allows a direct image of the body's energy to be seen on sensitive film, (Moss, 1979) has been found to be useful in detecting cancer. Probes are placed over the body, and changes in frequency and polarity of the corona around the body allow disturbances to be detected (Gerber, 1988). It is quite possible that, in the near future, medical diagnosis of internal events may be done by assessing the etheric energy field.

Coronal Discharge Photography

In the past two decades, Victor Inyuskin has demonstrated by coronal discharge photography that acupuncture points exist. He described the human energy field as a bioplasmic one composed of free ions, and likened it to a fifth state of matter. Balance of these minute particles is essential for health (Ostrander & Schroeder, 1977, p. 218).

COMPARISON OF SENSITIVES' PERCEPTION AND ELECTRONIC DATA

Another fascinating study of the human energy field was done by Dr. Valerie Hunt and others at UCLA in collaboration with the intuitive, Rev. Rosalyn Bruyere. While subjects were being treated with body therapy, several clairvoyants observed changes in the energy field that were recorded electronically. Mathematical analysis of the data showed consistent wave forms and frequencies that related to the auric colors and intensities perceived by the sensitive observer. So we now have further electronic indication of the presence of the human energy field and its associated colors (Hunt, reported in Bruyere & Farrens, 1989, pp. 247–259). The study concludes, "Throughout the centuries in which sensitives have seen and described the auric emissions, this is the first objective electronic evidence of frequency, amplitude and times which validates their subjective observation of color discharge."

Brain Wave Patterns in Healers

Puharich measured a life-enhancing alternating magnetic field, at an 8-hertz rhythm, emanating from healers' hands. In his observations, increased or decreased frequencies seemed detrimental to life. Dr. Robert Beck, a nuclear physicist, found that the brain waves of healers across many groups and cultures exhibit the same brain-wave pattern, 7.8–8 hertz, when giving healing. These energy patterns fluctuate with the earth's magnetic field resonance of 7.8–8 hertz, which are called *Schumann waves*. Healers' brains synchronize both in frequency and phase with the Schumann waves; this is called *field coupling*. This coupling appears to provide access to a large field of energy for the work of healing (Brennan, 1993, p. 18).

THE ENDOGENOUS HEALING PROCESS

Healing is mentioned in professional literature in limited ways, focusing primarily on the healer, healing techniques, and wound healing. Healing involves individuals in their own process. In other words, only clients can heal themselves. The author has observed six separate elements occurring in healing in which individuals move from disharmonious to harmonious patterns. These elements, which comprise the endogenous healing process, include:

1. Awareness
2. Appraisal
3. Choosing
4. Acceptance
5. Alignment
6. Outcome

Let's examine each of these aspects of the endogenous healing process (Scandrett-Hibdon & Freel, 1989) in more depth.

Awareness

Awareness is the alerting mechanism that cues individuals to events within their internal and external environments. The disturbance may be physical, emotional, mental, or spiritual and is often perceived internally by the client. The cue is sometimes a vibrational one to disturbances in the energy field. Awareness is critical to any healing process because if we are not aware of an issue, it cannot be addressed for change.

As an example of awareness, we consider the case of a client who was being interviewed and reported being aware of fatigue, irritability, and pain. She was aware that something was amiss because, in her own words, "I feel like I'm dragging, many times I'm barking at the kids, and I know for sure that something isn't right."

Appraisal

The second element in the endogenous healing process is appraisal. In appraisal, the individual explores and evaluates what awareness has brought to consciousness, assigns meaning to the disruption or cues, and makes comparisons with previous experiences, both from one's own knowledge and that of others. This knowledge may involve health information from a variety of sources.

To gain a greater understanding of appraisal, we look at the example of a physician who was also seeking help as a client. He knew something was wrong and tried to compare the symptoms with some of his previous experiences. He examined various syndromes of which he was aware and knew that this time his symptoms were different. He was using his expert knowledge to try to appraise the situation. After 3 to 4 weeks, when nothing shifted, he knew it was beyond the scope of his previous experiences and sought further medical and psychological help.

In other situations of appraisal, people know right away what the symptoms are and what to do. In these instances, they can go from awareness to appraisal and on to decision-making, basing the action on their appraisal.

Choosing

From appraisal emerges a sense of clarity with which one can choose and set goals to handle the disharmony. In choosing, a client often makes decisions quickly without focusing much energy on them, as though from the subconscious. Thus, the decision can be inferred by observing the client's actions rather than by waiting for a cognitive statement. Some individuals choose to use the disharmony as an opportunity to learn, and they consciously involve themselves in examining all of the life pattern implications of the illness. Some clients choose to avoid focusing on the disharmony altogether; still others allow the disharmony to run its course or simply choose to yield to its disturbance.

Acceptance

Acceptance might be considered to be a further aspect of choosing. In the process of "letting go," or deciding to accept, tension is released and relaxation occurs. With relaxation, energy shifts more easily so that repatterning to a more healthy state can occur with less effort.

In my research, acceptance can be readily seen in catastrophically ill individuals. For example, one young woman reported having double pneumonia with concurrent bacterial and viral infections. As she lay in intensive care and was responding poorly to her medical regime, she reported reaching a point in her illness where she simply released herself to her Higher Power, explaining that she felt it did not matter whether she lived or died. With this release, she began to heal more quickly and recovered fully.

Acceptance, then, is associated with making choices and yielding to changes. Three main characteristics of acceptance seem to apply: (1) giving in to what is occurring, (2) letting go or ceasing to fix the disturbance, and (3) surrendering or passing responsibility of control to another, such as to a health care provider or Higher Power. Nonacceptance, on the other hand, occurs with a "fight it off" stance or with denial that any disturbance exists.

Alignment

Alignment allows for the integration of the internal and external actions that support the movement toward harmony. In alignment, the energy shifts toward the goal of healing. Actions include activities such as changing one's diet, resting, or leaving uncomfortable situations. For example, a client stated, "To have ease in my life, I may need to leave a stressful job."

Outcome

The endpoint or outcome of healing is a sense of being in harmony and experiencing a sense of wholeness. Healing, like health and illness, is value related and defined by clients in their own terms (Barrett, 1990). Informants reported that they clearly knew when they were healed. Descriptors that might be anticipated with healing include physical and psychological comfort, vitality, a sense of peace, and an inner knowing of wellness. These findings are part of research studies of endogenous healing (Scandrett-Hibdon, 1988, 1989, 1990).

Model of the Endogenous Healing Process We can now look at a model of the endogenous healing process with the elements we have named in table 2.2.

AWARENESS
    physical cues
    emotional cues
    mental and spiritual cues

APPRAISAL
    evaluating
    comparing with previous learning
    assigning meaning to the disruption

CHOOSING
    setting goal

ACCEPTANCE
    yielding, turning it over, or nonaccepting

ALIGNMENT
    internal and external actions

OUTCOME
    harmony
    experience of wholeness

TABLE 2.2 Endogenous Healing Process

ENDOGENOUS HEALING COMPARED WITH ESTABLISHED SYMPTOM RESPONSE PATTERNS

As we examine the literature on human responses to illness and disharmonious patterns, we see two major models. One may be described as a symptom response model based on sociological studies of illness behavior (Chrisman, 1977; Kasl & Cobb, 1966; Suchman, 1965; Zola, 1964) and is characterized by the simple seeking of symptom relief. The other is more psychologically oriented and involves learning better coping skills. This approach is often encompassed in coping or stress management strategies (Cohen & Lazarus, 1973; Lazarus & Folkman, 1984).

Neither of these more established models has been compared to the actual healing process, which we now understand to be more integrative and client centered. In table 2.3 we compare the endogenous healing process with the coping model and the illness response model to note the differences. As we can see, the coping and illness response models report observed behaviors without exploring the client's inner experience, commitment, or participation. In other words, acceptance and the possibility of aligning with resources and action are missing. The outcomes, therefore, are also quite different.

SUMMARY

This brief history indicates a wide variety of human experiences with healing beyond mere symptom removal or coping with stress. The innate healing potential within the client needs to be honored by the facilitator who can help and assist the endogenous process that we have described. The transformational view of healing suggests that the client gains a new perspective through awareness, appraisal, choosing, accepting, and aligning.

Energetic interventions that work with the human energy field allow the sensitivity and respect for the client's choices that can foster activation of the healing potential. The history of energy-oriented healing ranges from simple "laying on of hands" to working with the human energy field and more sophisticated measurements of the aura as we have discussed in this chapter.

Endogenous Healing Process	Coping Model	Illness Response Model

Awareness
    physical
    emotional
	—	presymptom cue
		symptom recognition

Appraisal
    evaluate
    compare
    assign meaning
	cognitive appraisal
	adequate response
	    repertoire
	judgment
	discrimination
	choice of activity
		evaluation
		labeling
		monitoring

Choosing
    denial
    fight it off
    treatment
    let go
    inferred from action
	deployment of coping
	    mechanisms
		symptom definition
		social environment
		    for resources and
		    treatment

Acceptance	—	—

Alignment
    self-action
    others' actions
	recovery from stress	treatment of symptoms

Outcome
    harmony
    well-being
    peace
    vitality
	absence of stress	absence of symptoms

TABLE 2.3 *Comparison of Healing, Coping, and Illness Response Models*

We will explore energy field theory and its practical applications in part 2, but first we want to consider the most pertinent research related to energy-based healing. All of the history and research indicate we are yet at the very beginning of full understanding and investigation of this vitally important work.

References

Barrett, E. A. M. (1990). Health patterning with clients in a private practice environment. In M. Barrett (Ed.), *Visions of Rogers' science-based nursing*. New York: National League for Nursing.

Brennan, B. A. (1993). *Light emerging: The journey of personal healing*. New York: Bantam Books.

Bruyere, R., & Farrens, J. (1989). *Wheels of light: A study of the chakras.* San Madre, CA: Bon Publishers.

Chrisman, N. J. (1977). The health seeking process: An approach to the natural history of illness. *Culture Medicine Psychiatry, 1,* 351–377.

Cohen, F., & Lazarus, R. S. (1973). Active coping processes, coping dispositions, and recovery from surgery. *Psychosomatic Medicine, 35,* 375–389.

Elkin, A. P. C. (1978). *Aboriginal men of high degree.* New York: St. Martin's Press.

Gerber, R. (1988). *Vibrational medicine.* Santa Fe, NM: Bear and Company.

Grad, B. (1979). Some biological effects of laying on of hands and their implications. In Otto and Knights (Eds.), *Dimensions in wholistic healing: New frontiers in the treatment of the whole person.* Chicago: Nelson-Hall.

Hover-Kramer, D. (1993). *Energetic impressions of Egypt.* Poway, CA: Behavioral Health Consultants.

Kasl, S. V., & Cobb, S. (1966). Health behavior, illness behavior, and sick behavior: Part I. *Archives of Environmental Health, 13,* 246–266; Part II. Sick role behavior. *Archives of Environmental Health, 13,* 531–541.

Katz, R. (1982). *Boiling energy: Community healing among the Kalahari Kung.* Cambridge, MA: Harvard University Press.

Keegan, L. (1988). The history and future of healing. In *Holistic nursing: A handbook for practice.* Rockville, MD: Aspen Publishers.

Krieger, D. (1987). *Living the Therapeutic Touch.* New York: Dodd, Mead and Company.

Landy, D. (1977). *Culture, disease and healing: Studies on medical anthropology.* New York: Macmillan.

Lazarus, R. S., & Folkman, S. (1984). *Stress, appraisal and coping.* New York: Springer Publishing Company.

Moss, T. (1979). *The body electric.* Los Angeles: J. P. Tarcher, Inc.

Motoyama, H. (1981). A biophysical eclucidation of the meridian and Ki-energy. *International Association for Religion and Parapsychology, 7:1.*

Ostrander, S., & Schroeder, L. (1977). *Psychic discoveries behind the iron curtain.* New York: Bantam.

Pavek, R. (1993). *Manual healing methods: Physical and biofield* (Report). Washington, DC; National Institute of Health — Office of Alternative Medicine.

Rose, R. (1987, June 3). Magnetic pulses in RA: Less pain and mobility gain. *Medical Tribune.*

Rush, J. E. (1981). *Towards a general theory of healing.* Washington, DC: University Press of America.

Scandrett-Hibdon, S. (1988, February). *The endogenous healing process in elderly black women.* Study presented at second annual conference of the Southern Nursing Research Society, Atlanta, GA.

Scandrett-Hibdon, S. (1990). The endogenous healing process in adult women. *Journal of Holistic Nursing, 8*(1), 47–62.

Scandrett-Hibdon, S., & Freel, M. (1989). The endogenous healing process: Conceptual analysis. *Journal of Holistic Nursing, 7*(1), 66–72.

Shealey, N. (1979). Wholistic healing and the relief of pain. In Otto and Knights (Eds.), *Dimensions of wholistic healing: New frontiers in the treatment of the whole person.* Chicago: Nelson-Hall.

Stavish, S., & Horwitz, N. (1987, March 11). Pioneering cancer electrotherapy. *Medical Tribune.*

Suchman, E. A. (1965). Stages of illness and medical care. *Journal of Health and Human Behavior, 6,* 114–128.

Taubes, G. (1986). One electrifying possibility. *Discover.*

Veth, I. (1949). *The yellow emperor's classic of internal medicine.* Berkeley, CA: University of California Press.

Zola, I. K. (1964). Illness behavior of the working class: Implications and recommendations. In A. Shostak, & W. Gomberg (Eds.), *Blue collar work: Studies of the American worker.* Englewood Cliffs, NJ: Prentice-Hall.

3 | RESEARCH FOUNDATIONS

Sharon Scandrett-Hibdon, PhD, RN

What we touch with our hearts expands, heals, and grows.

Sharon Scandrett-Hibdon

INTRODUCTION

The purpose of this chapter is to review the literature and research related to energetic healing. We recall that throughout history an understanding of the human energy emanations, or biofield, served as a basis for various approaches used to help people in need. A number of energy-based approaches are currently gaining popularity because our highly developed medical technology requires the balance of human touch and intuitive perception.

THE HEALING TOUCH PROGRAM

Healing Touch is one such energy-based approach. Therapeutic Touch, Barbara Brennan's School of Healing Science, Rosalyn Bruyere's Crucible Program, and Pavek's Shen Therapy (Pavek, 1987) are other examples. Healing Touch involves a systematic approach to healing using energy interventions that incorporate a variety of therapeutic maneuvers. These will be presented in part 3.

The Healing Touch program, as it has been developed through the American Holistic Nurses' Association, offers a multi-level training experience that incorporates selected interventions to affect the human energy system. The Healing Touch program teaches basic elements of Therapeutic Touch; interventions described by Brugh Joy; concepts delineated by Rosalyn Bruyere and Barbara Brennan; and original techniques identified by Janet

Mentgen, the program originator, and her students.

MODELS OF TOUCH

As we begin to examine Healing Touch and the theoretical foundations, we find three philosophical models of touch. The first is a physical-sensory model that implies actual contact with one's body. The second is the psychological-humanistic model that involves a sense of caring for another person. The third is the field model involving interactions between individuals and their environments. Touch according to each of these models can mean, (1) to be in contact with, (2) to reach out, to commune with, and (3) to lay on hands, which means to overlap biofields (Weber, 1984). Since the third model most appropriately fits Healing Touch, we will explore it further.

FIELD MODEL

Rene Weber (1984) reminds us of the field model's power in examining Michelangelo's *The Creation of Man* painting in the Sistine Chapel. God is portrayed as a healthy, abundantly energetic organism stretching out a dynamic hand toward the limp and lifeless hand of Adam to transmit the spark of life. God deliberately and intentionally directs the energy to the depleted hand, yet these hands do not touch. So it is with many of the healing interventions. Energy is directed toward a client's depleted system to fill the human energy field and create buoyancy, health, and vitality.

Energy Exchange

What exactly occurs in the human energy field when there is an energy exchange? Many writers in energy-oriented work have attributed healing to an actual transfer of energy. Others speak of resonance that allows the client's field to pattern in new ways. Still others point to biochemical changes through enzyme and hemoglobin shifts that appear to result from energy exchanges. We will explore these possibilities citing some of the nearly 300 research studies that have been done in relation to healing without direct physical contact (Dossey, 1993, p. 200).

Transfer of Energy   Evidence of the electrical nature of the human body and communication within and around the body is mounting. Stravena (1991) reviewed research which provides evidence for the electrical nature of human beings and energetic communication for healing, particularly attempting to show that Therapeutic Touch may be an energetic form of communication. She reported evidence of electrical communication in fish and migratory birds by citing Hopkins (1977) and Warnke (1979). In the human body, the development of sensitive machines to measure energy fields which allow electrical fields in the myocardium (electrocardiogram), brain (electroencephalogram) and around the whole body (magnetogram) to be seen, was noted (Cohen, 1972; Swithenby, 1987). Next, evidence of the human aura or energy field (Kilner, 1965) and direct currents within the neural system which are believed to generate electrical signals forming a low–level electromagnetic field (Becker & Marina, 1982; Becker & Selden, 1985) was presented. This neural system may be the way the body detects tissue injury and heals; regulates sleep and wakefulness cycles; and responds to anesthesia, hypnosis, and biological rhythms. Further evidence is cited in Stravena's article on the electrical nature of the body in which conduction, electricity in bone and connective tissues, and biologically closed electrical circuits occur within the body (Cope, 1975; Norderstrem, 1983; & Thomsen, 1985). Low frequencies of electrical current have been used to stimulate neuronal cell differentiation and growth and for osteogenesis in bone fractures (Robinson, 1985). While this evidence is not conclusive, Stravena's review makes a strong argument for considering energetic communication as a means of energetic intervention.

Further evidence of the electromagnetic field is presented by Rubik (1993) who reports evidence of an ultraweak biological light emission, which may be explained biochemically or biophysically. The biochemical explanation views ultraweak biological light as an insignificant waste product of biochemical reactions. However, the biophysical perspective holds that biophoton emission is indicative of the innate electromagnetic field of the entire organism. Other researchers detail a photon emission theory in which the DNA molecule emits weak levels of radiation, which is speculated to be a rapid intercellular communication system (Peat, 1991; Popp, Li, & Gu, 1982; Rubik, 1993).

Wound healing, especially of pressure ulcers, has been accelerated by use of pulsed high peak power electromagnetic energy (Masdyoshi, 1991). Thus we see a mounting body of evidence that electrical phenomena exist within the body and may be one plausible explanation of healing through energetic approaches.

Energy Field Patterning   Many nursing writers use Rogers' theory, called the Science of the Unitary Human Being, as another explanation of what occurs in healing. In Rogers' theory the nurse is an integral part of the patient's environmental energy field patterning. The healing intervention is the "purposive patterning of energy fields in which the nurse uses his or her hands as a mediating focus in the continuing patterning of the mutual patient-environmental energy field process" (Meehan, 1990, p. 74). Change occurs in the human-environmental energy field as the nurse centers, connects with personal "unitary nature and integrality with the environmental field," and focuses on helping the patient. This interaction of the interconnecting fields, Rogers explains, is a "continuous mutual process of motion and change with each field reflecting the unique individual patterns." Thus, the nurse assesses the patient's field with the hands and helps direct the field to a more open symmetrical pattern that enhances the client's well-being. Meehan quotes Rogers in a personal communication as saying that our work is "to strengthen the coherence and integrity of the human and environmental fields and to knowingly participate in patterning of human and environmental fields for realization of maximum well-being."

Quinn (1993) captures this idea with a slightly different slant by saying that the Therapeutic Touch practitioner knowingly participates in the mutual human/environment process by shifting consciousness into a state of "healing meditation." This focusing of the healer's intention facilitates a repatterning of the recipient's energy through mutual resonance rather than energy exchange, allowing right relationship to emerge.

RESEARCH INTO ENERGY-BASED HEALING

Enzyme Studies

Research into energy-based healing began with the work of Bernard Grad of McGill University and Sr. M. Justa Smith of Rosary Hill College. Both studied the healing effect of Oscar Estebany who practiced laying on of hands for more than 25

Estebany who practiced laying on of hands for more than 25 years to demonstrate altered plant growth, wound healing in mice, and enzyme action (Grad, 1963, 1964; Smith, 1972). In general these early studies demonstrated that a healer's hands significantly affect growth and cellular repair in contrast to control and nonhealer groups.

Dr. Dolores Krieger's Studies Dolores Krieger built upon this early work by theorizing that enzymes affecting hemoglobin levels of erythrocytes may be influenced by laying on of hands. Hemoglobin, considered critical to oxygen transportation and sensitive to the individual's total state, was selected as index of change. Krieger hypothesized that a concomitant increase in oxygen uptake of the ill person would optimize metabolism with the laying on of hands. Forty-three chronically ill persons received healing treatments from Estebany, and 33 persons who accompanied the afflicted person served as the control group. Experimental subjects were treated daily, some twice daily. Hands were placed over the affected area with some subjects receiving light massage. Each subject was treated with purposeful intent on the part of the healer. Clients were also encouraged to rest for 30 minutes after treatment. Pretest blood samples were compared to final treatment post-test samples, with control samples drawn at the end of the study. Significant differences in pretest and post-test hemoglobin means were seen in the experimental group and between post-test means of experimental and control groups (Krieger, 1973). A second study repeated these findings, with control for factors thought to influence hemoglobin values such as smoking, yoga, and diet (Krieger, 1990).

Krieger then trained registered nurses in the laying on of hands technique of Therapeutic Touch (Quinn, 1988). She had 34 hospital patients receive Therapeutic Touch comparing results with 34 hospital patients receiving standard care. Pretest hemoglobin levels showed no significant difference between groups, whereas post-test group means showed significant increases in hemoglobin in the treatment group. This study, according to Quinn, still lacked operational definitions, random assignment to groups, and control for placebo and Hawthorne effects.

With Peper and Ancoli, Krieger examined physiological responses of the healer and the healee during Therapeutic Touch

(Krieger, Peper, & Ancoli, 1979). The healer was monitored by recordings of electroencephalography, electromyography, electrooculography, and galvanic skin, and patients were monitored for responses with these instruments as well as hand temperature. Krieger, the healer, was able to focus her attention continuously without effort or drifting into hypnogogic imagery and demonstrated an unusual amount of "fast syndrome beta activity." Three patients were reported to be quite relaxed with high amplitude alpha activity when their eyes were open and closed.

Relaxation Effects

Building on Krieger's findings about the physiological relaxation effects of Therapeutic Touch, Heidt (1979, 1981) studied the effect of this procedure on state anxiety of hospitalized cardiovascular patients. Three groups of 30 patients completed the A-State Self-Evaluation Questionnaire (Spielberger et al., 1970). Group A received modified Therapeutic Touch (5-minute procedure with 90-second modulation over the solar plexus), Group B received casual touch of 1-minute pulses (apical, radial, and pedal), and Group C had a nurse visit for 5 minutes with no touch. The A-State Self-Evaluation was readministered and comparison was made with pretest means. Statistically significant differences were seen only in the Therapeutic Touch group ($p > .001$) using correlated T ratios.

Janet Quinn's Research Using Therapeutic Touch   Quinn (1981, 1983) demonstrated similar results in a study in which non-contact Therapeutic Touch was compared to movements that mimicked Therapeutic Touch without centering, intention to assist the patient, attending to the patient's condition, or directing the energy. A 5-minute intervention of both procedures was used with 60 patients hospitalized in a cardiac unit. Again, acute anxiety on the State-trait evaluation instrument was significantly decreased in the treatment group ($p > .005$).

Later, Quinn (1989) utilized a 5-minute non-contact Therapeutic Touch process with a 120-second holding over the solar plexus in a replication study on pre-post open heart surgery patients. Mimic Therapeutic Touch and a no-treatment group were measured as well with no eye contact or monitoring of facial expression. Quinn delivered both the treatment and mimic group interventions. Included in the study were 153 patients hospitalized for open-heart surgery. Pre-post treatment assessments were made followed by a retention measure 1 hour later. Results using six separate analyses of covariance (ANCOVA) revealed no significant differences among groups, yet changes occurred in the expected direction. The Therapeutic Touch group did have significant reduction in diastolic blood pressure, which was not seen in the untreated group. One confounding variable for this study was that 72% of these patients were receiving calcium channel blockers or beta-andrenergic blocking agents or both. Another variable was that the investigator, an experienced Therapeutic Touch practitioner, delivered both the experimental and mimic touch interventions, which produced automatic behavioral responses to facilitate healing of the patient. Treatment times were greatly shortened from those used in the usual Therapeutic Touch procedures. The study also pointed to the need for more qualitative data from both the practitioner and the patient.

Randolph's Stress Studies Involving Therapeutic Touch

Randolph (1979) studied physiological aspects of stress (muscle tension, skin conductance levels, and skin temperature) and found no significant differences in two groups of college students treated with Therapeutic Touch and casual touch. Each subject was held on the lower abdomen and back for 13 minutes while watching a stressful film. The Therapeutic Touch practitioners centered, intended to assist the patient, and consciously directed energy to the subject whereas the untrained control nurses simply mimicked the hand positions. Treatment measurements were made 8 minutes into the film at the peak of stressful images, and findings between the treatment and control groups were not statistically significant. Several reasons for these findings were suggested: substantial deviation from usual procedure in administration of Therapeutic Touch, use of healthy subjects, and elicitation of a normal response to stressful stimuli may have produced some energy exchange.

Neonatal Therapeutic Touch Studies

Fedorik (1984) studied neonates to evaluate response to stress and found a significant reduction in infant state of arousal for the non-contact Therapeutic Touch group. In contrast, the mock Therapeutic

Touch and no-treatment groups showed no changes. In fact, infant arousal increased with the mock Therapeutic Touch group, which may signify normal infant responses to short stimulation. No significant differences were found for the transcutaneous oxygen blood gas pressure. There were methodological problems with this study in that the mimic treatments were not equivalent and measurement times varied.

Therapeutic Touch Studies with Elderly Hospitalized Patients   Another study on state anxiety was done with elderly hospitalized patients. Three groups were developed: one received a non-contact form of Therapeutic Touch, another received a mimic form, and a third group simply had a nurse holding closed hands over the patient's shoulder. Pre-post test scores of the A-State Self-Evaluation Questionnaire were analyzed revealing no statistically significant differences. One explanation offered was that this practitioner had only two years of experience in Therapeutic Touch, which was less than that of practitioners in other studies (Parkes, 1985).

Immune System Changes

In 1987 Quinn studied four bereaved people who were treated by two experienced Therapeutic Touch practitioners, each of whom offered clinically practiced protocols. A significant change in the immune system was seen in all four individuals with a reduction of suppresser T cells, whose function is to reduce or turn off activities of the immune system. Other measures of the immune system were not impacted. Participants reported reduction in state anxiety in half of the subjects following Therapeutic Touch and dramatic improvement in psychological variables, such as joy, vigor, and contentment (Quinn & Strelhaushas, 1993).

Pain Relief Studies

Keller found highly significant decreases in pain scores on the McGill-Melzack Pain Questionnaire of tension headache subjects treated with non-contact Therapeutic Touch, which differed from the mimic control group (Keller, 1983; Keller & Bzdek, 1986). In another study, postoperative pain in 108 adults did not show significant differences when Therapeutic Touch or mimic Therapeutic

Touch were used (Meehan, 1985). Pain scores on the Visual Analogue Scale and Pain Intensity Descriptor form were significantly lowered by standard treatment of intramuscular injection of a narcotic. The author used a rigorous analysis and a 5-minute treatment time that may have been insufficient for acute pain. However, later evaluation and secondary analysis by the same author indicated that the treatment group was significantly effective in lowering postoperative pain and also that patients waited longer before requesting more analgesia (Meehan, 1986).

Interventions with Children Boguslawski (1980) discussed the theoretical benefits of Therapeutic Touch in pain relief, which still need further research. A study comparing Therapeutic Touch and casual touch in stress reduction of 30 hospitalized children aged 2 weeks to 2 years revealed significant differences in the treatment group. Therapeutic Touch produced calmness and changes in pulse rate, peripheral skin temperature, and galvanic skin response ($p > .05$) (Kramer, 1990). Children were touched when the parents were not in the room and external stimuli were reduced. The casual touch consisted of stroking or patting on the head for 6 minutes, the Therapeutic Touch was given for 6 minutes. Measurements were taken 3 and 6 minutes after the interventions were completed. Children in the Therapeutic Touch group calmed down more quickly after stressful experiences such as medical procedures.

Interventions with the Elderly Fanslow, who has worked extensively with the human energy field in the elderly, found that patients with advanced arteriosclerotic heart disease responded to continuous, repetitive Therapeutic Touch on a daily basis with ambulation and mobility. When three of these subjects became bed-bound a year later, Therapeutic Touch prevented decubiti in two of the patients and also healed the decubitus of a patient that developed skin breakdown when on another nursing unit within 3 weeks. In a second study of four elderly osteoarthritic patients, pain as well as inflammation and joint swelling were decreased with Therapeutic Touch as the primary therapy. These changes were maintained for 1 year. In a third study, Fanslow treated eight stroke veterans, five with right hemiplegia and three with left-sided involvement. After 6 months of Therapeutic Touch treatment, pain and spasticity of affected upper extremities decreased appreciably. These changes occurred more quickly and lasted longer in right-sided hemiplegics. All of these patients reported that they felt a sensation of flow or movement in the affected extremity and experienced a reduction in fear and anxiety (Fanslow, 1984). In addition, three nurses reported that improved quality of sleep in five elderly nursing home patients seemed to be attributed to Therapeutic Touch (Braun, Layton, & Braun, 1986).

Preparation for Childbirth

Childbirth is another area being studied by Krieger (1979). Of particular interest is the impact of Therapeutic Touch on the couple's relationship. Pilot results indicate that Therapeutic Touch enhances couples' sharing and emotional support during delivery. Wolfson (1984) reports that Therapeutic Touch is effective in treating anxiety, discomfort, and complications of pregnancy and in fostering interconnectedness in families.

Accelerated Wound Healing

Therapeutic Touch has been found to speed wound healing. A dramatic reduction in wound size was seen in a randomized double blind study using non-contact Therapeutic Touch. Forty-four healthy male volunteers had a surgical biopsy done on the lateral deltoid muscle. Each subject came for a daily measurement placing his arm through a sleeve in the wall into a second room where the size of the wound was examined, and non-contact Therapeutic Touch treatments were done on half of the group. For the 16 days of the experiment, measurements indicated that on day 8 the Therapeutic Touch group had an average wound size 10 times smaller than that of untreated controls. By the end of the treatment period, the wound size was greatly diminished, with 23 of the experimental subjects having total wound healing, whereas none of the control groups showed complete wound closure (Wirth, 1991).

Patient/Healer Interaction

A qualitative study by Heidt (1990) focused on the experience of the healer as well as that of the patient. Seven nurses who practiced Therapeutic Touch from 3 to 11 years were solicited and paired with one of their patients whom they had treated from 10 to 100 sessions (median = 30). Each pair was observed and notes were made on all verbal and nonverbal behavior during the Therapeutic Touch session. Then each individual was interviewed and taped separately to recount what the process and experience of using Therapeutic Touch was like. The data was handled using a grounded theory methodology of coding and analysis. Key content areas that emerged were *opening intent,* which included affirming, quieting, and attending; *opening sensitivity,* which included attuning and planning; and *opening communication,* which included unblocking, engaging, and enlivening. Each of the nurses used all phases of the Therapeutic Touch intervention as described by Krieger (1979). Patients' experiences paralleled that of the nurses in sensing relaxation and calming.

Case Studies

In addition to the previously mentioned formal studies, various case studies with different populations are appearing in the literature. Use of Therapeutic Touch with rehabilitation clients, in helping patients to rest, for symptom reduction with AIDS patients, with mental patients, and for closure of a large wound — these are a few of the direct studies that are being published in the nursing literature (Heidt, 1991; Hill & Oliver, 1993; Newshan, 1989; Payne, 1989; Wetzel, 1993). A human energy field assessment form has also been developed and is being validated by Wright (1991).

FUTURE RESEARCH POSSIBILITIES

Several issues still need to be addressed. First of all, we might obtain a more accurate picture of the potential usage of Therapeutic Touch through a standardization of clinical interventions that more closely parallel procedures utilized in actual practice. As noted, most of the studies utilized a 5-minute intervention. In addition, modification of Therapeutic Touch with a simple hand-holding position does not really test what practitioners do. Length of treatment time is usually based on client need and the practitioner's intuitive perception.

Secondly, more double-blind studies or clinical trials are needed to see what is possible in the three areas most noteworthy in Therapeutic Touch — eliciting the relaxation response, reducing pain, and speeding healing. More qualitative studies are needed to provide greater understanding about this holistic intervention that enhances the personal wellness of the practitioner while simultaneously supporting the healing of the client.

SUMMARY

As seen in this review of literature, most of the current studies of energetic healing use Therapeutic Touch. Even though some studies are inconclusive the majority of research findings indicate three major effects: (1) rapid relaxation response, (2) amelioration or eradication of pain, and (3) acceleration of wound healing (Krieger, 1990). Krieger attributes relaxation to a "dampering of the autonomic nervous system" as seen by reduced blood pressure and respiratory rate and lowered pulse and pupil dilation in the peripheral nervous system. This response assists persons with asthma, paralyticileus, colic, gastrointestinal and genitourinary system spasms, secondary symptoms of AIDS, cancer, and cardiopulmonary and kidney problems. Psychosomatic stress-related disorders such as panic attacks, hysteria, and other hyperactive states are also alleviated. The second clinical change, a significant reduction in pain, may result in less need for medications. In addition, greater movement in painful musculoskeletal ailments and independent functions occur, mood is altered with heightened sense of well-being, and depression is decreased. Finally, acceleration of wound healing is noted. Fractured bones knit more quickly, and immune function is enhanced (Krieger, 1990, 1991).

References

Becker, R. O., & Marina, A. A. (1982). *Electromagnetism and life*. Albany, NY: State University of New York Press.

Becker, R. O., & Selden, G. (1985). *The body electric: Electromagnetism and the foundation of life*. New York: William Morrow.

Boguslawski, M. (1980). A facilitator of pain relief. *Topics in Clinical Nursing*, pp. 27–37.

Braun, D., Layton, J., & Braun, J. (1986). Therapeutic Touch improves residents' sleep. *American Health Care Association Journal, 12:1*, 48–49.

Cohen, D. (1972). Magnetoencephalography: Detection of the brain's electrical activity with a superconducting magnetometer. *Science, 175:4022*, 664–666.

Cope, F. W. (1975). A review of the applications of solid state physics concepts to biological systems. *Journal of Biological Physics, 3:1*, 1–41.

Dossey, L. (1993). *Healing words*. San Francisco: HarperCollins.

Fanslow, C. A. (1984). Touch and the elderly. In C. C. Brown & N. J. Skillman (Eds.), *The many facets of touch*. Brunswick, NJ: Johnson and Johnson, 183–189.

Fedorik, R. B. (1984). Transfer of relaxation response: Therapeutic Touch as a method for reduction of stress in premature neonates. Unpublished doctoral dissertation, New York University.

Grad, B. (1963). A telekinetic effect on plant growth. *International Journal of Parapsychology, 6*, 473–498.

Grad, B. (1964). A telekinetic effect on plant growth II. Experiments involving treatment of saline in stopped bottles. *International Journal of Parapsychology, 6*, 476–499.

Heidt, P. (1979). An investigation of the effects of Therapeutic Touch on anxiety of hospitalized patients. Unpublished doctoral dissertation, New York University.

Heidt, P. (1981). Effects of Therapeutic Touch on anxiety level of hospitalized patients. *Nursing Research, 1*, 32–37.

Heidt, P. (1990). Openness: A qualitative analysis of nurses' and patients' experiences of Therapeutic Touch. *Image: Journal of Nursing Scholarship, 22:3*, 180–186.

Heidt, P. (1991). Helping patients to rest: Clinical studies in Therapeutic Touch. *Holistic Nursing Practice, 5:4*, 57–66.

Hill, L., & Oliver, N. (1993). Technique integration: Therapeutic Touch and theory based mental health nursing. *Journal of Psychosocial Nursing, 31:2*, 19–22.

Hopkins, A. (1977). Electric communication. In T. A. Sebeok (Ed.), *How animals communicate*. Bloomington, IN: Indiana University Press (pp. 263–289).

Keller, E. (1983). The effects of Therapeutic Touch on tension headache pain. Unpublished master's thesis, University of Missouri.

Keller, E., & Bzdek, V. M. (1986). Effects of Therapeutic Touch on tension headache. *Nursing Research, 35:2*, 101–105.

Kilner, W. J. (1965). *The human aura.* New Hyde Park, NY: University Books.

Kramer, N. A. (1990). Comparison of Therapeutic Touch and casual touch in stress reduction of hospitalized children. *Pediatric Nursing, 16:5,* 483–485.

Krieger, D. (1973, March 21–23). *The relationship of touch with intent to help or heal to subjects' in-vivo hemoglobin values: A study in personalized interaction.* Paper presented at Kansas City, ANA.

Krieger, D. (1979). *Living the Therapeutic Touch: Healing as a lifestyle.* New York: Dodd, Mead.

Krieger, D. (1990). Therapeutic Touch: Two decades of research, teaching and clinical practice. *Imprint,* pp. 83–88.

Krieger, D. (1991). Therapeutic Touch: Toward an understanding of unitary human be-ness. *Cooperative Connection: Newsletter of Nurse Healers, 12:1,* 3–4.

Krieger, D., Peper, E., & Ancoli, S. (1979). Therapeutic Touch: Searching for evidence of physiological change. *American Journal of Nursing, 4,* 660–662.

Masdyoshi, I. (1991). Accelerated wound healing of pressure ulcers by pulsed high peak power electromagnetic energy (diapulse). *Decubitus, 4,* 24–32.

Meehan, M. (1985). The effect of Therapeutic Touch on experience of acute pain in post operative patients. Unpublished doctoral dissertation, New York University.

Meehan, M. (1986). The effect of Therapeutic Touch on acute pain secondary analysis. Unpublished report, New York University Medical Center, Department of Nursing.

Meehan, T. C. (1990). The science of unitary human beings and theory-based practice: Therapeutic Touch. In M. Barrett (Ed.), *Visions of Rogers' science-based nursing.* New York: National League for Nursing.

Newshan, G. (1989). Therapeutic Touch for symptom control in persons with AIDS. *Holistic Nursing Practice, 3:4,* 45–51.

Norderstrem, B. E. W. (1983). *Biologically closed electric circuits.* Stockholm, Sweden: Nordic Medical Publication.

Parkes, B. (1985). Therapeutic Touch as an intervention to reduce anxiety in elderly hospitalized patients. Unpublished doctoral dissertation, University of Texas at Austin.

Pavek, R. R. (1987). *Handbook of Shen.* Sausalito, CA: The Shen Institute.

Payne, M. B. (1989). The use of Therapeutic Touch with rehabilitation clients. *Rehabilitation Nursing, 14:2,* 69–72.

Peat, F. D. (1991, Autumn). Light and life. *Noetic Science Review*, pp. 24–25.

Popp, F. A., Li, K. H., & Gu, G. (Eds.). (1982). *Recent advances in biophoton research*. Singapore: World Scientific.

Quinn, J. (1981). An investigation of the effects of Therapeutic Touch done without physical contact on state anxiety of hospitalized cardiovascular patients. Unpublished doctoral dissertation, New York University.

Quinn, J. (1983). Therapeutic Touch as energy exchange: Testing the theory. *Advances in Nursing Science, 6*, 42–49.

Quinn, J. F. (1988). Building a body of knowledge: Research on Therapeutic Touch 1974–1986. *Journal of Holistic Nursing, 6*, 37–45.

Quinn, J. (1989). Therapeutic Touch as energy exchange: Replication and extension. *Nursing Science Quarterly*, pp. 79–87.

Quinn, J. (1993). Therapeutic Touch. *International Society for the Study of Subtle Energies and Energy Medicine Newsletter, 4:1*, 5–6.

Quinn, J., & Strelkauskas, A. J. (1993). Psychoimmunologic effects of Therapeutic Touch on practitioners and recently bereaved recipients: A pilot study. *Advances in Nursing Science, 15:4*, 13–26.

Randolph, D. (1979). The difference in physiological response of female college students exposed to stressful stimuli when simultaneously treated by Therapeutic Touch or casual touch. Unpublished doctoral dissertation, New York University.

Robinson, K. R. (1985). The responses of cells to electric fields. *Journal of Cell Biology, 101:6*, 2023–2027.

Rubik, B. (1993, Summer). Natural light from organisms: What, if anything, can it tell us? *Noetic Science Review*, p. 15.

Smith, J. (1972, Spring). Paranormal effects on enzyme activity. *Human Dimensions*.

Spielberger, C. D. (1970). *STAI manual for the state-trait anxiety inventory*. Palo Alto, CA: Consulting Psychologists' Press.

Stravena, J. E. (1991). Therapeutic Touch: Placebo effect or energetic form of communication. *Journal of Holistic Nursing, 9:2*, 41–61.

Swithenby, S. J. (1987). Biomagnetism and the biomagnetic problem. *Physics in Medicine and Biology, 32:1*, 3–4.

Thomsen, D. E. (1985). Electrifying biology. *Science News, 127*, 268–269.

Warnke, U. (1979). Information transmission by means of electrical biofields. In F. A. Popp, (Ed.), *Electromagnetic bio-information*. Munich, Germany: Urban and Scheuartenberg.

Weber, R. (1984). Philosophies of touch. In C. C. Brown & N. J. Skillman (Eds.), *The many facets of touch. The foundation of experience, its importance through life with initial emphasis for infants and young children.* Brunswick, NJ: Johnson and Johnson.

Wetzel, W. (1993). Healing Touch as a nursing intervention. *Journal of Holistic Nursing, 11:3.*

Willborn, S. N. (1987, March 30). An electrifying new hazard. *US News and World Report,* pp. 72–74.

Wirth, D. (1991). The effect of non-contact Therapeutic Touch on the healing rate of full thickness dermal wounds. *Journal of Subtle Energies, 1:1.*

Wolfson, I. S. (1984). Therapeutic Touch and midwifery. In Brown & Skillman (Eds.), *The many facets of touch.* Brunswick, NJ: Johnson and Johnson, 166–172.

Wright, S. M. (1991). Validity of human energy field assessment form. *Western Journal of Nursing Research, 13:5,* 635–647.

2 THE HUMAN ENERGY FIELD

*I*n this part we will explore the nature of the human energy field, the seven major energy centers and their properties, and the implications of these concepts for assessment by the healer.

FIELD THEORY AND IMPLICATIONS FOR HUMAN CARING

4

*Consciousness is sometimes compared to a light, and
different bodies, to the lampshades which cover it.
These shades surround the light, one inside the other,
each of a different color and material. Each shade
captures light to a certain degree and is illuminated by
it. Each transforms the light and modifies it according
to its properties. . . . Each shade fits inside consciousness. Each is denser than the one just interior to it. . . .
Because of the way these bodies cover up and conceal
the underlying consciousness they are often called in
the ancient philosophical writings 'sheaths.'*

Rama, Ballentine, & Ajaya, 1981

*The concept of field provides a means of perceiving
people and their respective environments as irreducible wholes.*

Rogers, 1991

INTRODUCTION

Of all the health care professions, nursing has perhaps the best-
defined concept of itself as the art and science of human caring.

A number of nursing theorists (Rogers, 1970; Watson, 1985) have written extensively about caring as a central quality in the profession. Of course, all health care professionals share the basic desire to help those in need and to facilitate a caring relationship between helper and client. A unique aspect of nursing, however, is its concern for the promotion of health and well-being taking into account the environment that is in constant interaction with individuals and their groups. This concern led nursing theorist Martha Rogers (1991) to develop her concepts of the irreducible nature of individuals as energy fields integral with the environmental field. We will explore the basis of this theory in current understandings of physics and human relationships and see how the use of noninvasive, energetic modalities flows from Rogers' theoretical model.

THE FIELD CONCEPT

As helping professionals, we are often aware that the relationship between helper and client becomes the vehicle for healing, rather than the use of a specific procedure or method. We rightly become curious about what really occurs in a healing interaction. It seems there is creative sharing that occurs even in the most subtle and simple caring event (Watson, 1988). Something genuine is exchanged between the caregiver and the patient. We might call this intuition, the sensing and knowing of a client's needs, due to the interpersonal communication skills of the helper. More specifically, we can use the Rogerian model that suggests there is an exchange or influencing resonance between the human energy fields. In this model, the healer emits a vibration or frequency to which the client responds, often entirely outside of his cognitive awareness. We will explore this model in more detail, since it underlies our basic knowledge of energy-based approaches (like Healing Touch and Therapeutic Touch) in health care.

The Energy Field as Part of Human Environment

As we discussed in chapter 2, the concept of an energy field that is part of the human interactive environment is as old as recorded history. Ancient Indian traditions, more than 5,000 years old, speak of a universal energy called *prana* that flows in relation to the spine and activates the life force, or *kundalini*. This breath of life moves through all living forms and can be enhanced by breathing techniques, meditative practices, and the specific techniques of yoga. The Chinese called this basic life energy *ch'i*, which exemplified balance in a healthy person. An imbalance of this energy force could result in physical illness. In the Kabbalah of Jewish mysticism this energy was called the astral light. Throughout the last two millennia artists have depicted halos around Christian saints to signify their expanded energy and enlightenment. The quality of increased energy was called *spiritus* in Latin, and is the root of the English word spirit, or soul. Although the ability to actually see the energy seemed to be available only to a few initiates or advanced students, all persons could sense the heightened energy in a teacher or leader and respond to it.

To this day, we use a variety of phrases that incorporate energetic concepts into our thinking patterns. For example, when we are in the presence of someone who is especially high in energy and awareness, we say we feel "charged," "in tune," "energized," or that the "vibrations are harmonious." When we spend time with a person of low energy, we feel "drained" or "depleted" of our own vitality. As we study human energies, we recognize that these are not merely metaphors or poetic descriptions but accurate depictions of what occurs at the energetic, *pranic*, or *ch'i* level.

Nonphysical Events   Other experiences that we share as human beings point to the reality of nonphysical events, occurrences that go beyond our understanding of the material plane. Telepathy, precognitive dreams, and the sense of influencing each other, especially loved ones, over vast distances suggest there is some connection between individuals beyond physical presence. More than 70% of Americans have had some experience of expanded consciousness and extrasensory perception, including the more than 8 million persons who have had near-death experiences (Gallup, 1982; Ring, 1984). This is all the more remarkable when we consider that most people in our culture are highly materialistic and concrete in their worldview.

If we allow ourselves to see the mind as a hologram that extends beyond the narrow constraints of space and time, we can understand the existence of these phenomena better (Pribram, 1979, pp. 71–84). In the holographic model, information about the whole is encoded in every part, just as a single musical tone has all other tones embedded in it and allows us to hear the harmonics in the overtones several octaves above. Or, to use another approach, we seem to have a local mind tied to immediate facts and events that is encompassed within a larger, nonlocal mind that allows us to sense our interconnectedness with others (Dossey, 1991). The soul, which is the nonlocal manifestation of our expanded consciousness, senses the interconnection with others through means that extend well beyond our physical bodies. It appears, then, that we are interconnected with each other in highly complex and subtle ways: what we do and think influences everything else and affects the whole.

Interactive Fields   One way that we can understand these interconnections is through the concept of interactive *fields*. Fields bring objects separated by space into relation with each other. In the past hundred years, the idea of a field to describe an invisible and nonmaterial emanation from an object has come into use in scientific terminology. For instance, the electromagnetic envelope generated by a dynamo is called its electromagnetic field. Increasing scientific evidence, especially from quantum mechanics, holds that all bodies, from the atom and subatomic particles to the great earth itself, have their own fields, whatever size they may be (Capra, 1977, p. 196).

More than a hundred years ago, the well-known British physicist, Faraday, saw with intuitive perception the lines of stress or "force fields" surrounding magnets and used this perception to describe the action of electric currents in space (Capra, p. 47). Faraday also sensed that the entire universe is made up of these force field lines and perceived light as electromagnetic radiation long before science could prove the nature of light as wave and particle. What Faraday sensed at the intuitive level was later proven mathematically and empirically to be correct.

The animal kingdom makes good use of the reality of energy fields in stalking prey. Sharks and rays, for instance, have electroreceptors that aid them in finding future meals, as all living organisms emit electromagnetic vibrations and have an energy field. Recent findings suggest that some mammals also use electroreceptors in settings where vision is limited, as in the case of the burrowing "electric" mole (Zimmer, 1993, p. 16). It appears, then, that the energy field is a fundamental underlying unit of all matter and is especially prominent in living systems.

THE HUMAN ENERGY FIELD

Moving up the evolutionary ladder, we can recognize that there is an energy field that surrounds, flows through, and extends from the human body. It is undoubtedly more complex than that of the animal kingdom and can be sensed with the development of our higher sense perceptions. In ancient times, this emanation was called the *aura* and was perceived by mystics and clairvoyants as a visible phenomenon. We are now able to measure this energy field, or human energy emanation, with delicate scientific instruments. The Japanese physicist Motoyama has developed a number of electrode devices that actually measure the human bioelectrical field at various distances from the surface of the body (Motoyama, 1984, p. 257).

We can have increasing appreciation for the sensitives and clairvoyants who accurately described human energy fields long before scientific confirmation was available. With tools only of higher sense perception of subtle energies, clairvoyants like Dora Kunz (Karigulla & Kunz, 1989) were able to diagnose complex medical problems by sensing the client's energy field and noting "fullness" or "emptiness" in relation to parts of the body. In his work as a physicist, Motoyama "found strong correlation between meridians that are electrically out of balance and the presence of underlying disease" (Motoyama, 1984, p. 257). Thus, it is now possible to clinically assess a person's energy field to determine where there is an excess or lack of energy as a way of learning about a client's state of health. *Vibrational Medicine* (Gerber, 1988) is a fascinating book that captures the essence of this new energy-based approach and its implications for medical practice.

It is not so much that we *have* an energy field but rather that we *are* an energy field of which the physical body is the most visible and dense. The field essentially remains the same, whereas the material "stuff" of which we are made is constantly changing. Like a river that is consistent in shape but ever changing in content, the human body changes its cellular and molecular structure daily. Linings of the intestinal tract change every 3 to 4 days; other tissues replace and repair themselves in a few weeks (Chopra, 1991, p. 48). We know the physical body to be more than 85% water, but even the molecules of water are 99.99% space as we understand the conclusions quantum physicists draw about the nature of the spaces between subatomic particles. Within the energy field, protein and water molecules vibrate synchronously to influence ganglia, nerve plexuses, blood composition, endocrine secretions, and a multitude of other body processes. Emotions and thoughts vibrate within the field as well and may serve to transmit feelings and information to other human fields.

Layers of the Energy Field

Let us move on now to the specific layers of the human energy field and how they create a new understanding of ourselves and what may occur during a healing session. Many texts, both ancient and modern, describe the various layers, sheaths, or bodies of the energy field (Kunz & Peper, 1985; Leadbeater, 1980).

The Work of Dora Kunz   For nursing and the healing professions, Dora Kunz is best known as the gentle and persistent influence behind Dr. Dolores Krieger's development of Therapeutic Touch at New York University. Together they pioneered the development of the first modern, energy-based therapy and brought their knowledge to students throughout the world. Although many texts discuss the possibility of seven or more layers in the energy field, for our discussion we will use Kunz's four-level description. Her framework gives many insights about functions of the field layers and implications for assessment and intervention.

According to Kunz, these are the four major layers or dimensions of the energy field of most direct significance for healing work (Kunz & Peper, 1985, pp. 213–261):

1. The vital layer, also sometimes called the *etheric field*, is most closely associated with the physical body and interfaces with the emotional dimension. It extends 2 to 12 inches from the skin and is the layer most associated with energy-balancing healing work.

2. The emotional layer, sometimes loosely called aura in older texts, extends further than the etheric field, and holds the individual's affective, feeling energy.

3. The mental layer, still further from the skin, embodies our thinking patterns and visual imagery. It is often called the *causal layer* in ancient texts.

4. The intuitive layer is sometimes called the *astral body* and relates to the spiritual dimension of the individual.

Other layers of the energy field that have been observed are the etheric template, the celestial body, and the ketheric body, which constitute the physical, emotional, and mental aspects in the more subtle planes (Brennan, 1987, p. 47).

Sensing the Energy Field As the energy field of the client is sensed, the nurse or healing professional can assess the state of the energy. Lowered energy in the vital field, for example, is often the precursor of physical pathology. This state may be experienced by the client as irritability or fatigue. Often, field assessment with the hands can detect dysfunction before it actually becomes physical illness or more severe exhaustion. This suggests the great value of energy-based modalities in giving early feedback before symptoms become evident in the physical body. The ability to detect impairments for early screening and prevention is thus one of the greatest gifts of the energy field therapies.

IMPLICATIONS FOR PRACTICAL APPLICATION

The recognition of the human being as a multidimensional field with energy as its dynamic force holds many implications for healing work. The mechanistic view of the body as a machine with replaceable parts gives way to the vision of each of us as a total human being who is at all times interconnected with the environment. Each human interaction now can be viewed as an exchange of energy between two interacting fields, as figure 4.1 shows. From this image we can appreciate the need to approach the energy field of a client with care and awareness.

Another concern is awareness of our own field as caregivers. With practice and intentionality we can learn to be sensitive to

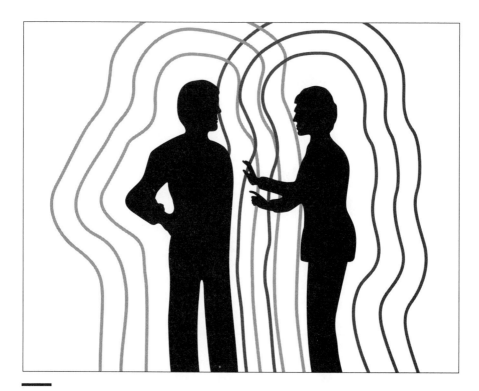

FIGURE 4.1   Human interaction seen as an energy exchange of the two fields.

areas of depletion or imbalance and learn how to remain in the best possible state of health. When we see the impact of the two energy fields on each other, we know there is no way to hide our internal state in the physical, emotional, mental, or spiritual dimensions. At best, therapists or healers can recognize that their attitudes, beliefs, and opinions are communicated in many, often subliminal, ways. As psychotherapists have come to recognize, communication is a multilevel process, and we may not even know which part of our subconscious qualities reaches the subconscious of the client (Bandler & Grinder, 1975). Increasing our self-awareness and self-healing capacity is, therefore, our most important goal. This will be explored in depth in the last part of the book.

Working with the Energy Field Layers

As we look at the client, we come to see that imbalance or dysfunction may occur in any of the layers of the energy field. To use the four-dimensional pattern we discussed earlier, we can now picture in figure 4.2 the interactive layers, each one enfolded in the next in a hierarchic fashion. Each successive layer encompasses more of the whole than the previous one, although they are probably not as separate or discrete as the diagram suggests. Seeing the layers of the energy field also shows us the reasons that removal of a physical problem, as by surgical procedure, is

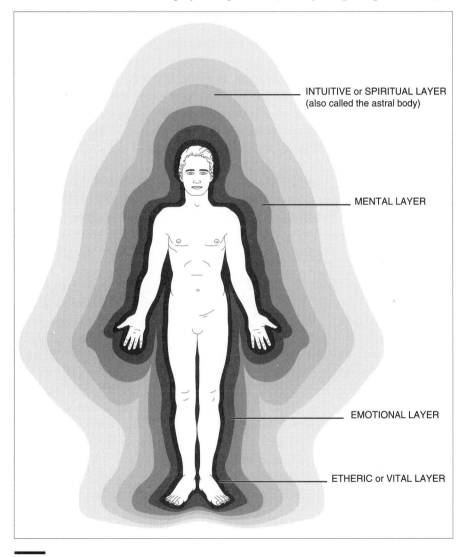

INTUITIVE or SPIRITUAL LAYER
(also called the astral body)

MENTAL LAYER

EMOTIONAL LAYER

ETHERIC or VITAL LAYER

FIGURE 4.2   Four major layers of the human energy field extending beyond the physical body (other layers are also seen but are more subtle).

often not sufficient to bring balance and harmony to the entire system. To put it another way, the body is influenced by the emotions, the mind, and the spiritual consciousness of the individual. The mind, connected to Infinite Intelligence, is much more complex than the body, the emotions, or the thoughts by themselves and encompasses or enfolds all of them.

As we see the model of the successive layers of the energy field, we observe that dysfunction in the spiritual, or intuitive, layer is undoubtedly the most devastating because it impacts all other layers. It is no accident that the great psychologist, Carl Jung, declared that the most significant disease of the twentieth century is loss of meaning and spiritual disconnection (Jung, 1964). Dysfunction in the spiritual layer is experienced as a loss of purpose or sense of hope in one's life. Dysfunction in the mental layer is manifest in faulty thought patterns and self-doubt. Dysfunction in the emotional layer relates to constricting affect, such as depression or despair. Dysfunction or blockage of energy flows in the physical dimension, and the related vital layer, can result in physical symptoms and disease.

This way of thinking leads us to understand most physical disease as the end stage of a much longer process. Recent exploration into the adult onset of cancer, for example, suggests that the actual tumor development occurs within 1 to 3 years after a significant loss or shock (Simonton, Mathews-Simonton, & Creighton, 1981, pp. 47–64). Initially, the individual loses a sense of purpose or meaning in life. The universe no longer seems friendly or hope-inspiring. Then, negative thought patterns begin to take form and predominate, such as "I can't make it" or "life is not worth living." In time, depression and other negative emotions take over. The dysfunction in the three outer layers may be present, then, prior to the onset at the cellular level of a progressive disease such as cancer.

Another way that physical problems develop quickly is by traumatic injury. It is important to remember that all the layers are affected, that the entire energy field is jarred by trauma or accident, not just the vital layer. Treatment, similar to the long-term disease process, requires working from the innermost layer of the field to the outer layers. In the case of surgical intervention, a rebalancing of all the layers of the field is needed to complete the healing process, as we shall explore in chapters on healing interventions.

CONSIDERATIONS FOR HEALING

Therapeutic Touch, the best-known energy therapy in health care, is an easily learned approach for recognizing deficiencies in the energy field of the patient and for balancing the energy by interaction with the healer. As in more complex energy therapies, the healer reaches out from the energy field within herself to the vital or etheric energy field that surrounds a client's body. Actual physical touch does not seem to be important initially for balancing of the field. Later, a laying on of hands to modulate the energy is part of the Therapeutic Touch process.

The exact dynamic behind the healing of the energy fields is not yet well understood, but, as described in chapter 3, the effects of the healing interaction are measurable and significant. Applications of energy field therapies in psychotherapy also show that significant emotional changes can be effected by working directly with the energy field. This will be described in chapter 14.

Alignment with Higher Power

Another important implication of energy field theory for the healer is alignment with Higher Power or the Universal Energy Field (Brennan, p. 37), as the individual understands it. The healer does not drain his own strengths and resources to help someone else. Rather, he is a conduit for the universal life energy, the Source, or Higher Power. Burnout among healers is not possible if we are continually tapping into this limitless energy supply via our centering work. A sense of feeling drained or exhausted suggests that the healer may be attempting to use her own ego power instead of trusting the universal flow. Energy seems to move or resonate from the person with more energy to the person with depleted energy, from the stronger vibration to the weaker vibration, and to move the depleted pattern to a higher frequency. Therefore, it is essential that the healer be attuned to the higher vibrational frequencies and release as much tension or negativity as possible before reaching out to others.

SUMMARY

In essence, then, an energy-based, noninvasive approach such as Healing Touch is the application of the principles of energy balancing to the multidimensional field of the client. It appears there is an extension of energy from the Universal Energy Field through the healer to the client. To put it succinctly in computer language, there is input from the Universal Field, throughput of energy within the healer, and output to the client. The resonance that occurs in the interacting fields creates significant outcomes, bringing about significant changes in the physical, emotional, mental, and spiritual dimensions as we will explore in succeeding chapters.

References

Bandler, R., & Grinder, J. (1975). *Patterns of the hypnotic techniques of Milton Erickson* (Vol. 1). Cupertino, CA: Meta Publications.

Brennan, B. (1987). *Hands of light.* New York: Bantam Books.

Capra, F. (1977). *The Tao of physics.* New York: Bantam Books.

Chopra, D., MD (1990). *Quantum healing.* New York: Bantam Books.

Dossey, L., MD (1991). *Recovering the soul.* New York: Bantam Books.

Gallup, G. (1982). *Adventures in immortality.* New York: McGraw-Hill.

Gerber, R. (1988). *Vibrational medicine.* Santa Fe, NM: Bear and Co.

Jung, C. G. (1964). *Man and his symbols.* New York: Doubleday and Co.

Karigulla, S., & Kunz, D. (1989). *The chakras and the human energy fields.* Wheaton, IL: Theosophical Publishing House.

Kunz, D., & Peper, E. (1985). Fields and their clinical implications. In D. Kunz, (Ed.), *Spiritual aspects of the healing arts.* Wheaton, IL: Theosophical Publishing House.

Leadbeater, C. W. (1980). *The chakras.* Wheaton, IL: Theosophical Publishing House. (Original work published in 1927)

Motoyama, H. (1984). *Theories of the chakras.* Wheaton, IL: Theosophical Publishing House.

Pribram, K. (1979, February). Holographic memory. *Psychology Today.*

Rama, S., Ballentine, R., & Ajaya, S. (1981). *Yoga and psychotherapy.* Honesdale, PA: Himalayan International Institute.

Ring, K. (1984). *Heading toward omega: In search of the meaning of the near-death experience.* New York: William Morrow.

Rogers, M. E. (1970). *An introduction to the theoretical basis of nursing*. Philadelphia: Davis Publishing Co.

Rogers, M. E. (1991). Nursing science and the space age. *Nursing Science Quarterly, 5:1*, 27–34.

Simonton, C., Mathews-Simonton, S., & Creighton, J. L. (1981). *Getting well again*. New York: Bantam Books.

Watson, J. (1985). *Nursing: The philosophy and science of caring*. Boulder, CO: Colorado Associated University Press.

Watson, J. (1988). *Nursing: Human science and human care*. New York: National League for Nursing.

Zimmer, C. (1993, August). The electric mole. *Discover Magazine*.

5 | THE CHAKRAS AND THEIR FUNCTIONS

If one is to explore the world of inner experiences, his thoughts, his emotions and learn about himself, he must have some framework in which to do this. He must have a 'playroom' — a sort of workshop or laboratory in which he can experiment. . . . The framework provided by understanding the centers of consciousness (chakras) gives him a place to do this. It provides the student with a structured inner space in which he can play.

Rama, Ballentine, & Ajaya, 1981

INTRODUCTION

As we have seen, the human being is made up of a wondrous complex of layers or sheaths, starting with the physical body as the densest part and extending outward to form the dimensions of the entire energy field. Now we turn to another facet of the field, the concentrations or vortices of energy, called *chakras* from the Sanskrit word for wheel. These points of focus for energy were seen by the ancients as vortices of color and light, spinning at various speeds and influencing the entire field. Thus, they were appropriately named *wheels of light and energy.* In ancient as well as modern times, the chakras are understood as the receptors for the inflow of energy from the Universal Energy Field and the gateways to consciousness. They appear to mitigate communication between the various layers of the field and to ensure that energy flows to all parts of the human energy system.

THE CHAKRAS

Many writings describe the chakras, from Hindu and Sanskrit texts that form part of yogic practices (Tansley, 1985) to the lovely clairvoyant visions of the American theosophists of the early twentieth century (Besant & Leadbeater, 1925). The great sleeping prophet, Edgar Cayce, described the energy vortices and their relation to physical ailments, giving specific cures for each dysfunction that was presented to him (Reilly & Brod, 1975). More recently, the work of transpersonal psychotherapists (Small, 1982) incorporates chakra theory into psychological awareness. And, to top off a large array of references, we have the dynamic, fully illustrated writings of Rosalyn Bruyere (1989) and Barbara Brennan (1987).

Most of the material provides consensual agreement that the chakras exist and significantly influence the physical body as well as the emotions, mental patterns, and spiritual awareness. However, a great deal of diversity exists about specific facts, such as the particular functions of the physical body that are related to each chakra. Therefore, we are choosing for this discussion to follow the classical interpretation of Alice Bailey (1978, p. 45). Her work, which has been known for 50 years now, makes a definitive statement about complex body-mind interactions, and perhaps best exemplifies the cross-cultural orientation that is needed to comprehend the chakra system.

To allow scientific inquiry its due, we turn again to the Japanese researcher Motoyama. A lifelong student of yoga, he became intrigued with the origins of knowledge about the energy field. After confirming the existence of acupuncture meridian flows through electronic measurements, he confirmed the presence of the chakras in relation to seven major areas of the body along the outline of the spinal column (Motoyama, 1984).

Many other smaller energy centers exist and are called minor chakras. For the present, we will concentrate on the seven major centers and their fascinating impact on our human energy field.

LOCATION AND FUNCTION OF THE CHAKRAS

The following exploration of the chakras and their relationship to the energy field is based on extensive reading and the author's personal experience of working with the energy centers for more than 15 years. We will discuss the relation of each energy center to the body, to specific physiological functions, and to its influence on the endocrine glands. We will also consider the impact of the chakras in the psychological, mental, and spiritual dimensions to learn of the complex interrelationships that occur within the energy system. Figure 5.1 will help in understanding the

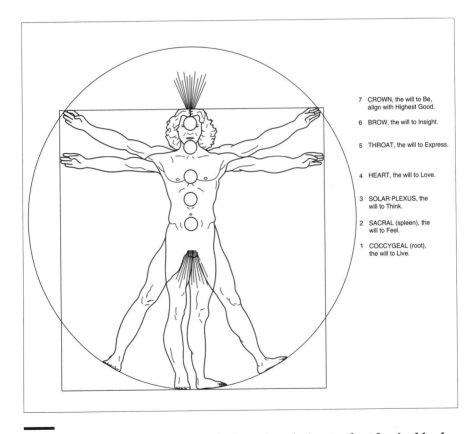

7 CROWN, the will to Be, align with Highest Good.

6 BROW, the will to Insight.

5 THROAT, the will to Express.

4 HEART, the will to Love.

3 SOLAR PLEXUS, the will to Think.

2 SACRAL (spleen), the will to Feel.

1 COCCYGEAL (root), the will to Live.

FIGURE 5.1 *The seven major chakras in relation to the physical body.*

Reprinted with permission from Janet L. Mentgen, Program Administrator, Healing Touch actual location of each energy vortex and its relation to the spinal column in the physical dimension of the energy field.

The Root or Coccygeal Chakra

The root or base chakra is located at the base of the spine and radiates downward from the perineal area of the body. Its location below the coccyx gives it the name most frequently used. In the yogic tradition it is the *muladhara*, the manifestation of life energy. The color of bright, clear red is associated with the relatively slow vibration of this center, and a motor or bumblebee captures its sound.

This center is related to the lower parts of the body — feet, legs, hips — and to functions of elimination and movement. Psychologically, this center is most related to our sense of belonging on the earth, feeling a sense of security, and having the will to survive and be fully alive. The adrenal glands, which sit on top of the kidneys, most influence this center through the body's survival responses. The fight/flight reaction, stimulated by adrenal excitation, is the body's animal-like ability to generate physiological peak performance to ensure survival. Physiological and psychological distress generating fear and worry can constrict the energy of this center. The long-term stresses of our society, in which the adrenals are constantly agitated, can cause immeasurable physical and emotional damage as can be seen in functional hypertension and anxiety states.

The will to live and to enjoy life is one of the greatest signs of optimum functioning of this chakra. As the body and mind are in close connection with each other, affirming mental patterns expands the energy flow through this center. Examples of life-affirming thoughts are "I feel my energy," "I am glad I am alive," "I am safe and secure; the universe is friendly." The related emotions are a sense of vitality, enthusiasm, and joy. The natural capacity to dance and move are physical expressions of this energy.

The Sacral Chakra

The sacral chakra, sometimes called the spleen center in ancient texts, is located halfway between the base of the spine and the end of the sternum, or just below the umbilicus. In the Indian texts this *svadhisthana* chakra is also related to the vital body energy and life force. The gonads, the endocrine glands of sexuality and reproduction, are associated with this center. Other related bodily functions are balance and assimilation of body fluids and absorption of nutrients through the large intestines.

Psychologically, this center is related to the expressions of sexuality and choosing appropriate relationships. Most of the addictive processes that so plague our culture appear to have their origins in this center and rob it of its vitality. Many addictions, we are now learning, are actually caused by poor chemical assimilation of foods that, in turn, impacts other layers of the energy field. For instance, the long-term effects of chemical imbalance in the physical field can cause irritability and create the wish to escape the intensity of physical and emotional pain. The pain can further be numbed by using addictive chemicals. Emotional imbalance and faulty thinking patterns develop over time to justify or rationalize this escape mechanism and become evident in other layers of the field as blocks in the energy flow.

The color that exemplifies the sacral center is orange, and the melody of a wooden flute evokes its sound. Seeing options, making choices, and being responsible for one's actions characterize healthy functioning of the center. Emotional qualities include the abililty to use all of one's resources and available energies appropriately. In the mental layer of the energy field, this center enables us to discriminate between helpful and unhelpful influences and to release unwanted thoughts and ideas. When the center is activated in positive ways, relationships with others fall into place easily, and we are able to readily utilize and integrate new information.

The Solar Plexus Chakra

Also called the *manipura*, this chakra is associated with power, strength, and the ability to feel one's ego identity. It is located near the solar plexus at the base of the sternum. The pancreas functions in this area by assisting in the digestion and storage of glucose. Physical distress, such as stomach ulcers, hypo- and hyperglycemia, and digestive disturbances of various kinds can be traced to blockage in the field around the third chakra.

Emotionally, this center relates to issues of control. People who have strong ego demands and dominate others represent an imbalance or distortion of this chakra. On the other hand, persons who are unduly passive or, worse yet, passive-aggressive also demonstrate imbalance of this center. Healthy psychological manifestation of this center is in assertive behavior. The words that best express these patterns are "I trust my ability to communicate," "I communicate effectively," "I feel my strength and respect others' strengths." As this center relates to the ability to use ego awareness and intellect effectively, it represents the will to think.

The color of the solar plexus chakra is the one that literally aids mental functioning — clear, lemon yellow. The sweet sound of stringed instruments represents the musical essence. Esoteric literature reports this center to be a storage battery for extra energy to use in difficult times. It is the center associated with staying power, the ability to start things and bring them to completion. Masculine and feminine aspects within each of us are balanced and harmonized through the ability to give and to receive, which has its power in the solar plexus chakra.

The Heart Chakra

The heart chakra, also called the *anahata* in the Indian tradition, is located at the center of the chest, between the nipples. The qualities of the heart center are those of harmonizing, loving, accepting love, and forgiving. The energy conveyed by this center is markedly different from that of the lower three that deal with the more material, earthbound work of ensuring survival, dealing with emotions, and thinking clearly. To put it another way, the lower centers address the physical, emotional, and mental dimensions as exemplified in the will to live, the will to feel, and the will to think. The heart center speaks from our soul level and is therefore associated with the will to love.

The color of life and hope, emerald green, is related to this center, and it is often described as the transformative center. The radiating sound of bells gives the auditory vibration of the heart center's energy. It serves to mitigate the earthbound energies of the lower three centers with the subtle, higher centers of the spiritual or intuitive dimensions. The thymus gland, a small endocrine gland now understood as a major stimulus of the immune system, relates to the physical dimension of this center. Associated physiological functions are the respiratory system and all parts of the cardiovascular network.

Heart center dysfunctions are plentiful at this time in history as heart disease and circulatory disorders are the leading cause of death in the West. The second leading cause of death is immune system dysfunction, either deficiency as in cancer and AIDS or overactivity as seen in the autoimmune diseases.

The heart is the seat of emotions we describe as love although we need to be careful to distinguish the kind of love we are discussing. Many popular song lyrics espouse a possessive emotion, more like the addiction and control of the second and third chakra areas, as love. The love of the heart center is a pure, spiritual caring, the essence of the thirteenth chapter of 1 Corinthians, verses 4, 5, 7, and 8 in the Bible: "Love is patient and kind; love is not jealous, or conceited, or proud; love is not ill-mannered, or selfish, or irritable; love never gives up: its faith, hope and patience never fail. Love is eternal." In short, the heart represents unconditional love and forgiveness.

When psychological work is done to release grudges, old hurts, and to forgive others, the energy of this center expands, which causes our immune system to become more active. Thought patterns for this center are "I forgive others easily," "I can give and receive unconditional positive regard," "I am loved and accepted by Universal Love." When we operate from the heart center and express devotion and service without internal conflicts, our true spiritual selves begin to emerge.

The Throat Chakra

The throat center is located in relation to the middle of the neck and influences the thyroid gland. In the yogic tradition, the *vishuddha* is the center of creative energy. As its location suggests, it relates to the throat, neck, esophagus, and the function of making sounds by singing or speaking. Perceptions of the senses, communication, self-expression, and beginning intuitive awareness emanate from this center.

Those who have activated the throat center with the full support of the lower centers speak in a rich, sure tone of voice and enjoy expressing themselves in written and spoken communication, delighting in the sharing of ideas. Dysfunctions of the center are evidenced by constrictions of the voice, hoarseness, frogs in the throat, and the holding back of creative ideas. Poor self-image is another manifestation of fifth center blockage. When we believe others always know more than we do, there is no sense of trust in ourselves or self-esteem.

The colors of turquoise or light blue express the vibration of the throat center as does the sound of wind blowing through the trees. Clairaudience, the ability to hear intuitively, begins to emerge when this center is open. The capabilities associated with this chakra are the communication of one's talents, knowledge, and understanding, affirming "I enjoy expressing who I am." Needless to say, it takes a commitment to personal growth over many years to achieve the sense of purpose that is exemplified by the will to express oneself confidently.

The Brow Chakra

As we continue to explore the finer, more subtle energies of the higher centers, we come to the brow chakra, often called the *ajna* center or the seat of the "third eye." Located in the middle of the forehead, this center is associated with the pituitary or master endocrine gland and is the focus of insight, vision, psychic awareness, clairvoyance, sentience, and the ability to sense nonphysical realities such as energy fields or auras.

As we might deduct, this center relates to the brain, eyes, ears, head, and nose in the physical dimension. Higher level thinking, mental processing, and sensory perception are other concomitants. In the emotional dimension, this center relates to a sense of self-identity, personal insight, and compassion for others. Mentally, when this center is active and open, there is a quality of knowing with wisdom, as opposed to mere cognition. The individual can evaluate and perceive accurately without judgment or prejudice, and unusual events are understandable from this expanded perspective.

Deep indigo blue is the color most often connected to this chakra and its sound is that of waves crashing on the beach. Increased ability to visualize and to receive mental imagery comes to us when this center is open and flowing. The willingness to see with insight and intuition or to put oneself in another's place characterizes this center. Another quality is the ability to combine unconditional love with wisdom.

Distortions of this center occur when a person taps into this energy without the grounding of the other centers. This is evidenced in the many persons who have New Age insights but use the information for selfish purposes or take a part of their experience to represent "the path" and impose it on themselves or others. Judgments and prejudicial thinking are another distortion of this level of consciousness.

The Crown Chakra

The crown chakra, the *sahasrara* center, is located above the middle of the head where the fontanels are joined. It is understood as the spiritual center, the center of connection with the wisdom and oneness of the universe. The colors associated are white, orchid, lavender, or purple according to different traditions. The sound that best symbolizes this center is the universal, harmonizing tone of "om" or "aum." The center may also be understood as the unifying principle of all color into white and of all sounds into the rainbow of full orchestral music.

As this is the highest energy vortex in relation to the physical body, it is the center of spirituality and soul-consciousness. Love, openness, a sense of purpose and expansion beyond the ego personality, and alignment with Higher Power are the qualities of this center. The will to be and the will to do whatever is for the highest good are manifest through the open crown chakra. In many traditions, headdresses, crowns, and halos signify the person who is actively using this center to give spiritual leadership to others. Another beautiful symbol is the thousand-petaled lotus that gives an image of divine beauty and complex simplicity. Often, when a person feels the energy of this center, there is a unitive glimpse, a sense of oneness and interconnectedness with all creation, and a brief understanding of ways in which everything is unified and whole.

The pineal gland, which sits just above the pituitary, is the endocrine gland associated with the crown center. The actual physiological functions of this gland are just being researched and appear to be related to the sense of timing that guides bio-rhythms, bodily functions such as the onset of puberty, and our responses to the seasons and sunlight (Tamarkin, Baird, & Almeida, 1985, p. 714).

Seen as the seat of the soul, the crown center has no major dysfunctions since we are always in connection with the Source of Life. We may at times limit the inflow of vital energy from the Universal Energy Field by our limited thinking or blockage in the emotional or physical energy flows of the other centers. The words that capture the essence of the crown chakra are "I am whole," "I am one with the universe," and "We are all interconnected."

Some sensitives attuned to higher sense perception report the presence of chakras above the crown. These may be considered extensions of the crown chakra that connect us more actively with nonlocal aspects of ourselves. As we tap into the dimensions beyond our personal selves, the transpersonal or more-than-personal aspect is activated. This seems to be our human interface with the wider, more expanded dimension of consciousness that is currently being explored in the field of transpersonal psychology.

RELATIONSHIP OF THE CHAKRAS TO THE ENERGY FIELD

In addressing the complexities of the chakra system, we are given an extraordinary and powerful tool for understanding human nature. We may wish to view the whole system as a useful metaphor for systematically tracking various aspects of body, emotions, mind, and spirit. Figure 5.2 helps us to visualize the chakras as they are felt: cone-shaped wheels of energy extending from their locations near the spinal column through the ever finer layers of the energy field, in both the front and back of the body.

As we combine the various qualities of each chakra and its relationship to the four major layers of the energy field, we can imagine a comprehensive chart, as in table 5.1 (see pages 70 and 71), to show the optimum functioning of each chakra. Knowing the optimum functions allows us in the healing profes-

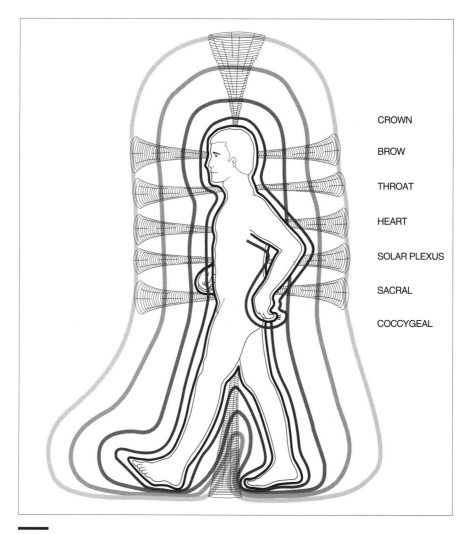

FIGURE 5.2 *The chakras in relation to the layers of the energy field.*

Reprinted with permission from Janet L. Mentgen, Program Administrator, Healing Touch

sions to spot deviations that could indicate early stages of dysfunction. We will also be able to make comparisons between relative states of wellness and the various dysfunctions to identify areas for healing work.

If we summarize the dysfunctions in relation to each center, we can trace the impact of imbalance on the physical,

Chakra	Physical	Emotional	Mental	Spiritual
Coccygeal or Root	Vital life energy flow Full enjoyment of being alive	Realistic and appropriate trust Responds with appropriate emotions to life events	"I am secure." "I belong on the earth." "I deserve to enjoy my life fully."	The universe is friendly.
Sacral	Fluid assimilation, elimination, and balance Sexual enjoyment	Positive self-image Able to sort out relationships and establish close bonds	Discrimination of positive and negative "I choose; I select." Able to release unwanted thoughts	Everything is open to choice. Cocreation
Solar Plexus	Good digestion and utilization of nutrients Muscles in harmony "Bounce" in walk	Balance of masculine and feminine aspects of personality Flexibility Sense of direction	"I am in charge of my life." "My energy is steady to accomplish my goals."	Work with laws of attraction

TABLE 5.1 *Optimum Function of Each Chakra and Related Field*

Chakra	Physical	Emotional	Mental	Spiritual
Heart	Sense of well-being Lightness, radiance in appearance Good posture	Forgives easily Able to send and receive love Feeling of satisfaction	"I am lovable and capable." "I forgive easily."	Awareness of the reality of the soul Radiant love
Throat	Full, rich sound in voice Creativity	Enjoys expressing self Willing to take risks Effective communication	Values own and others' ideas Enjoys sharing and teaching	Expresses soul's nature and purpose
Brow	Open, alert appearance Perception of details, beauty	Compassion for others Insight Sensitivity Sense of humor	Evaluates without judging "I see clearly." Plans ahead	The universe makes sense.
Crown	All energy centers open and flowing Body systems in harmony	Kinship with others Concern for all of human kind Joy and deep feelings	"I am one with the one." Higher sense perception	Mystical experiences Unitive glimpses merging with divine will

TABLE 5.1 *continued*

psychological, mental, and spiritual aspects of the energy field. These dysfunctions can be sensed by the practitioner of Healing Touch as areas of energy blockage or depletion experienced as coolness or absence of vibration. Or there may be a congestion of energy, a bulge of heat, experienced as imbalance on assessment. The blockage may affect only the outer dimensions of the field signifying spiritual disconnectedness, or it may reach into the mental dimension in the form of faulty thought patterns. In the emotional dimension, constrictions in the chakra field imply negative attitudes and feelings that may become part of a personality pattern or mood disorder over time. Finally, blockage may affect the physical body in the form of symptoms of disease. Table 5.2 (see pages 73 and 74) shows the major dysfunctions in each related layer of the field as a simple guide for the healing practitioner.

Another useful assessment tool is to sense the condition of each chakra individually. Alice Bailey (1978, p. 81), describes five major conditions of the chakras in her somewhat metaphorical style:

1. CLOSED, still and shut, yet with signs of life, silent and full of deep inertia.

2. OPENING, unsealed, and faintly tinged with color; the life pulsates.

3. QUICKENED, alive, alert in two directions; the two small doors are open wide.

4. RADIANT and reaching forth with vibrant note to all related centers.

5. BLENDED they are and each with each works rhythmically. The vital force flows through from all the planes.

These poetic descriptions from a great clairvoyant teacher give us some idea of the excitement of determining the state of each center. As we identify the state of the chakra — closed, opening, quickened, radiant, or blended — we can relate each center to its impact in the energy field. Further assessment of the field as a whole gives us an energy-based and intuitive perception of what is occurring with the client.

Chakra	Physical	Emotional	Mental	Spiritual
Coccygeal or Root	Fatigue Lack of body awareness Ailments of low back, hips, legs, perineum	Apathy Lack of energy, intensity, vitality Fear	Poor concentration Confusion Lack of motivation Passivity	Lack of purpose, meaning, or direction in life.
Sacral	Fluid imbalance Edema Chemical dependency Sexual disorders	Gullibility Greed Defensiveness Sexual disorders	Difficulty differentiating positive and negative Poor relationship skills	Victim consciousness Belief in fate Predetermination
Solar Plexus	Tension in muscles Addictions Stress disorders Digestive problems	Competitive Driven Compulsive Perfectionistic Domineering	Controlling Power-hungry Unable to trust others "I'm the only one who can do it right."	Aloneness No trust in Higher Power
Heart	Chest pain Stooped posture to protect heart Cardiovascular disease Immune disorders	Guilt Resentment Holding grudges Sorrow Loneliness	"Others should make me happy." "No one can love me enough."	Karmic indebtedness Trapped — no way out Have to earn love

TABLE 5.2 Dysfunctions in Each Chakra and Related Field

Chakra	Physical	Emotional	Mental	Spiritual
Throat	"Pinched" voice tone Hoarseness Throat problems	Unexpressive Poor self-esteem Closed, dull Unwilling to risk	"If I express myself, something terrible will happen." "Others are better than me."	"Universe is unfriendly and unsafe.
Brow	Visual, sensory problems Sinus and headache problems Difficulty with details	Poor insight Difficulty putting self in others' place	Rationalistic Concrete thinking Literal Critical and judgmental	God is judgment There is a great critic out there
	Minimal dysfunction as we are always connected to the Universal Energy Field. Some dysfunctions observed:			
Crown	Poor assimilation from UEF	Constricting emotions	Limited thinking "I don't deserve the best."	Disconnected View of God as too small and impersonal

TABLE 5.2   continued

CHAKRA MEDITATION

Progressing upward starting from the base of the spine:

Chakra 1
My mind is firm
And steadfast like a rock.
I am secure, and safe
Able to withstand all shock.

Chakra 2
My body energy flows at my command,
Emotions balanced, Mastery is in my hand.

Chakra 3
I rise to meet obstacles —
My path is clear.
I trust my guidance
Control is here.

Chakra 4
What can hold, constrict, or encumber me?
Nothing of this world: I am free. I am free!

Chakra 5
Awake! My sleeping powers within, Arise!
Like the wind in the trees, God's power within me lies.

Chakra 6
My soul flows
On waves of cosmic light.
My insight expands,
Intuition is right.

Chakra 7
My silence is an expanding wave
Of cosmic light —
Above, below, without, within,
To the left and to the right —
Everywhere
The universe lives within my peace.

SUMMARY

As we become more at ease in determining chakra and energy field interactions, we begin to notice certain patterns within each individual, almost like a psychic signature. In the next chapter we will explore the implications of these patterns for the work of understanding the client's needs. The selection of actual healing techniques can be made effectively when the healer has a good knowledge and skill base in assessing and understanding the functions of the chakras. We will explore specific applications of this knowledge in the third section of the book, which provides a wide variety of techniques for healing.

References

Bailey, A. (1978). *Esoteric healing*. New York: Lucis Publishing Co.

Besant, A., & Leadbeater, C. W. (1925). *Thought forms*. Wheaton, IL: Theosophical Publishing House.

Brennan, B. (1987). *Hands of light*. New York: Bantam Books.

Bruyere, R. (1989). *Wheels of light*. Arcadia, CA: Bon Productions.

Motoyama, H. (1984). *Theories of the chakras*. Wheaton, IL: Theosophical Publishing House.

Rama, S., Ballentine, R., & Ajaya, S. (1981). *Yoga and psychotherapy* (p. 217). Honesdale, PA: Himalayan International Institute.

Reilly, H. J., & Brod, R. (1975). *The Edgar Cayce handbook for health*. New York: Macmillan Publishing.

Small, J. (1982). *Transformers*. Marina Del Rey, CA: DeVorss and Co.

Tamarkin, L., Baird, C., & Almeida, O. F. (1985). Melantonin: A coordinating signal for mammalian reproduction. *Science, 227.*

Tansley, D. V. (1985). *Subtle body*. New York: Thames and Hudson.

ASSESSING AND IDENTIFYING PATTERNS IN THE ENERGY FIELD

The interweaving of the three fields of the personal self, together with their vehicle, the physical body, gives us a picture of human life which can be compared to a moving four-dimensional tapestry, whose warp and woof are composed of threads of differing qualities and textures and whose patterns shift and change as they cut across the path of time. The key to understanding the complexity of this process of interaction lies in its dynamism, for life is always characterized by growth and change.

Karagulla & Kunz, 1989

INTRODUCTION

The imagery of the interweaving energy dimensions suggests that there are distinctive patterns unique to the consciousness of each individual. As the healer begins to assess the distinctive layers and the state of each chakra, she can image an outline while doing a hand scan that gives a profile of the individual's energy field. This feedback from the field allows the healer to quickly identify a pattern of personal characteristics related to the individual. After the assessment is complete, one can make some inferences between the energy pattern and predominant psychological and physical issues presented by the client.

The healer uses the knowledge gained from understanding the functions of the chakras and their condition to make a holistic, integrative evaluation of the client. The healer's own preparation for this work is increasing self-awareness through centering and meditation, which we will discuss more thoroughly in later parts of this book.

IDENTIFYING THE PATTERNS IN THE ENERGY FIELD

The word *intuition* is derived from the Latin *intueri*, which means to consider or look within. True intuition is the function of a person who has developed higher levels of consciousness through daily attention to meditative practice. As the intellectual knowledge of the energy system and the wisdom of the higher sense perception combine, the healer can become highly perceptive and quickly identify needs of the client.

In this chapter we will explore some of the energetic patterns that can readily be perceived with experience and training. This discussion is naturally not intended to label any particular client as we see all persons as evolving, dynamic entities. The emphasis here is to understand and integrate information received from the sample energy fields described.

Effect of Blocked Chakras

As we discussed in the previous chapter, the chakras are the receptive points that allow the inflow of energy from the Universal Energy Field. If this receptor is blocked for any reason the client may be receiving an inadequate supply of supportive life force and may develop a depletion of energy in the physical or emotional dimensions that are associated with the chakra's functioning. Over time, a compensation for this depletion may develop in the form of an accumulation of energy, or overabundance, in another energy center. Like the genetic code that is inherent in every cell through the RNA and DNA molecules, the imprint of one or more closed, blocked chakras creates a pattern throughout the entire energy field. By way of analogy, consider how the motif, or basic theme, in music is repeated and integrated throughout an entire composition. We can also speak of certain basic patterns in the collective human psyche that are repeated and developed in each individual's lifetime. Jung called these archetypes. These concepts help us to understand how embedded constrictions of the energy field can be carried by the client for many years unless there is intentional correction or repatterning.

ASSESSING THE ENERGY FIELD

Learning to sense a client's energy field requires clarity, centering, development of our intuitive talents, and much practice. We are speaking here of the sensing of subtle vibrations that have just recently been found to be measurable by sensitive scientific technology. There will be no claps of thunder or neon lights; each therapist learns to define a way of sensing energy that is relevant to her cognitive thinking style.

All of the perceptive senses can come into play as the healer develops ways of describing fine and subtle energies. However, the caregiver may initially need to rely on her predominant perceptual system. We begin new learning from our point of comfort and our favorite way of talking about experience (Bandler & Grinder, 1982). Thus, a predominantly visual person would begin to "see," looking for the nuances and shadings around the client's physical body. Some highly skilled visual healers learn to see the colors of the aura, differentiating areas of darkness or light in relation to each chakra. On the other hand, an auditory individual might begin to sense areas of harmony and disharmony by picking up sounds in the energy field. Most healers are highly kinesthetic and are very comfortable with sensory perception through the hands. Some become very adept at distinguishing areas of fullness around an open chakra and areas of absence of this fullness suggesting a closed or obstructed chakra.

To use another description, the healer may sense warmth or a tingling vibration in a radiant, open center and coolness and less tingling in a closed center. Whatever mode of accessing sensory data is initially used, the healer learns to add the other perceptual systems to get a wide range of feedback from the client. Thus, the vibrational patterns of the energy field are accessible through our own learning of higher sense perception. Practice, and plenty of it, with relatively healthy persons to contrast with someone who is ill, is the best teacher.

Whatever means of assessment are used, the hands of the healer are the tools. The compassion of the healer is the perceiver. The mind of the healer is the interpreter. And the spirit or soul of the healer is the guide.

Documentation

A method or system of noting each observation is important. Symbols for the condition of each chakra can be used, such as a period for a chakra that is completely closed and circles of varying sizes to describe the degree of opening and intensity of the spin of the chakra, which is clockwise in a healthy chakra. It is also useful to make a visual representation or profile of the entire energy system. This assists us in recognizing significant patterns that relate to physical and emotional issues.

PHYSICAL PROBLEMS AS PATTERNS IN THE ENERGY FIELD

Immune System Deficiency

One current major illness that depletes the immune system is AIDS, Acquired Immunodeficiency Syndrome. The AIDS epidemic has mandated that we understand the immune system and its dysfunctions more fully. Here, a complex and often mutating retrovirus attacks the body's major immune cells, such as the T-4, and destroys them, leaving the victim subject to a vast array of opportunistic infections. In fact, AIDS sufferers do not die from the action of the virus but from the effects of some otherwise innocuous organism, such as the *Pneumocystis carinii*, that takes over when the body's usual defenses are missing.

Other physical illnesses also cause depletion or a shutting down of the immune system with an impact on the energy field. Chronic infections with long-term side effects or overexposure to environmental pollution overrides the defenders of the body. Cancer, the unchecked growth of abnormal cells, is another disease that drains and deprives the body of its immune resources.

Immune system deficiency has devastating effects on the energy field and the vitality of the individual. This deficiency in the field can be sensed by the Healing Touch therapist as an emptiness, a flatness, or lack of "bounce," especially in the lower centers. The higher centers — throat, brow, and crown — may often be overactive to compensate for the lack of vitality in the lower centers. We sometimes call this predominance of the mental centers "running on mental energy," which is a very apt description of what happens energetically.

Figure 6.1 suggests a way of mapping an immune deficiency pattern that was sensed by the hands of the healer in the etheric or vital field of an AIDS patient. The lack of energy can often be sensed in the emotional and causal fields as well. Knowing the basic pattern and its effect can guide the therapist to implement ways of bringing vitality back through hands-on techniques like the Full Body Connection, which we will describe in the next section.

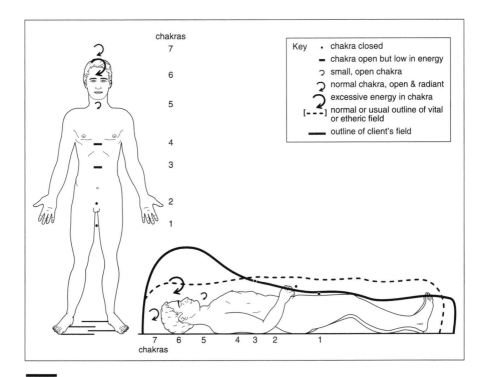

FIGURE 6.1   *Energetic pattern of immune system dysfunction.*

Autoimmune Diseases

A wide variety of physical dysfunctions, called autoimmune diseases, result from an overabundance of immune responses. In this instance, the systemic immune response is excessive and certain cells actually begin to attack the body. Examples of autoimmune diseases are lupus erythematosus, rheumatoid arthritis, some demyelinizing syndromes, and severe allergic reactions leading to asthma attacks. Chronic Fatigue Syndrome is currently understood as an autoimmune disease in which the body responds to viral and environmental stresses by being "on" all the time, thus depleting the endocrine glands, the thyroid and adrenals particularly, and exhausting the client's physical resources.

In the case of autoimmune disease, the therapist may hear the client describe symptoms of fatigue, achiness, and vague distress with a complementary lack of vitality in the entire energy field. A client with this problem will take on energy rapidly with laying on of the healer's hands, resulting in a sense of well-being and relief. However, this may only last a few minutes as the individual is unable to store the energy. It is helpful in autoimmune diseases to teach a family member or significant other how to facilitate maintaining energy balance. Eventually, through repeated working with the energy field, the client learns to maintain a steady flow of supportive and life-sustaining vitality. Over time this may permit a repatterning of the field toward balance and wholeness.

Cardiovascular Problems

As heart disease is the leading cause of sudden, unexpected deaths in the United States, energy field assessment is valuable in picking up early warning signals. In heart disease, the imprint of a chakra's diminished functioning can be noted in the emotional and mental dimensions of the field. This change in energy levels can be sensed well before physical symptoms, like angina or left quadrant pain, appear prior to a full-blown heart attack. As a matter of fact, many medical practitioners are beginning to note early warning signs in the emotional dimension by obtaining a full history of the client's lifestyle pattern.

The Type A Personality The Type A personality (Friedman & Rosenmann, 1974) is characteristic of an individual who learns to protect an emotionally wounded heart by overcompensating in other areas of life. Typically, this person feels driven to achieve, pushing herself and others unmercifully. This person may be a leader in her company who is domineering and compulsive, or a tyrant in her family. As others move away, she may push harder, which only drives others to further avoidance. The real need — to be loved and accepted unconditionally — is unmet and the person may feel embittered and alone.

From an energetic point of view, the Type A personality presents an overabundance of energy in the solar plexus chakra. This can also be apparent in the emotional and mental dimensions of the energy field, and the heart chakra may be weakened or closed. Often, the lower centers dealing with trust levels, survival issues, and sexual expression are depleted or shut down whereas the mental processes, especially the brow center, predominate as if to compensate for the missing pieces.

Figure 6.2 shows the profile of a counseling client who fit this personality pattern. Because he was in the early stages of its onset,

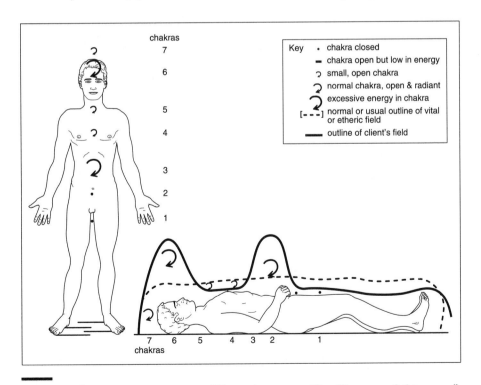

FIGURE 6.2 Energy pattern of Type A personality ("successful person" in our culture).

coming in for marital problems initially, much could be done to assist him in making lifestyle changes. By working through early childhood and career issues, he was able to reactivate the full function of the blocked centers and to achieve emotional harmony in his life. A good physical examination was imperative to check for possible physical damage, such as hypertension or circulatory disorders, and to begin a program of health awareness.

We begin to see, then, how assessment of a pattern can give the clue to needed lifestyle changes in the physical, emotional, and mental aspects toward balance of energy. This repatterning of the entire energy field appears to result in increasing levels of wellness and health.

High Stress Patterns

High levels of stress and emotional pressure are so prevalent that it is almost redundant to remind clients that stress may be affecting their sense of vitality and the energy field as a whole. It is usually easy to detect the signature of distress in the energy field if there is an absence of other physical symptoms. Constriction or closing of the root chakra is an obvious sign. The adrenals, which are programmed to respond to aversive stimuli, become overactive as pressure and the feeling of being threatened accumulate. When the adrenals have had too much stimulation, the body takes over with compensatory mechanisms, such as high blood pressure, that become generalized and systemic (Selye, 1978).

In figure 6.3 we see the profile of a young woman whose boss constantly harassed her. Her wish to do well kept her in this untenable position until she developed panic attacks and nightmares, which led her to seek counseling. The root chakra was completely blocked, and she expressed fear that she might not live long; her very survival was being threatened by the work situation. She attempted to compensate by trying harder, which caused an overexertion of the solar plexus, and by trying to be unconditionally loving, which taxed the heart center.

Fortunately, the emotional needs drove her to seek appropriate help before the problems led to physical disease. Many individuals can be helped by learning to relax, activating autogenic responses, and practicing biofeedback (Green & Green, 1977). Changes in lifestyle patterns can further help the client to relieve distress and, ultimately, to bring the energy field to higher balance.

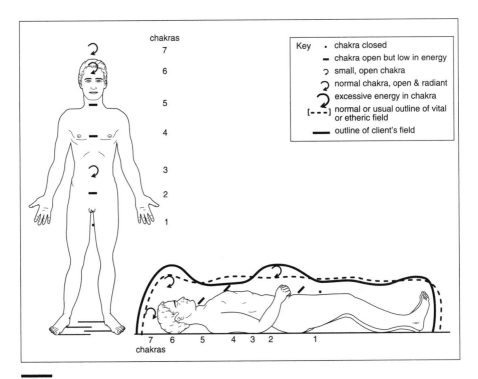

FIGURE 6.3 **Energy pattern related to high stress.**

Medical practitioners usually see persons with more advanced symptomatology — high blood pressure, headaches, glaucoma, adrenal or kidney dysfunctions. From an energetic point of view, we can see why just treating the condition with medication would be insufficient. Beyond lifestyle changes and health education, the individual must find ways to increase the inner sense of security and of safety, to open the root center, and to allow a full flow of energy to all the higher centers.

EMOTIONAL ISSUES IN THE ENERGY FIELD

Grief and Depression

Although grief and depression are predominantly emotional symptoms, they also have physical symptoms that most people recognize. Grief is a natural, emotional response to the loss of a loved one. As such it is not an abnormal state, although many individuals are surprised at the wide variety of strange thoughts, emotions, and physical symptoms that can occur. A healthy expression of grief diminishes over time and the individual can begin to reconnect with family and friends in new ways. An unhealthy grief reaction is one that persists over time (often well over several years), does not diminish in intensity, is denied, or is incapacitating to the individual.

Grief has a distinctive energetic pattern in which all the lower centers are diminished or blocked for a period of time with a concomitant loss of enjoyment of life and lowering of libido. Figure 6.4 shows the energy field profile of a client who was newly widowed with two young children in her charge. Needless to say, her entire world was upside down and shattered. She needed to literally

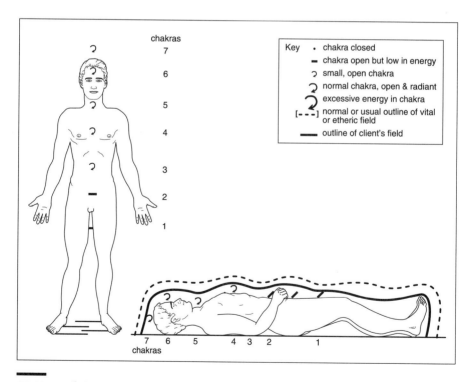

FIGURE 6.4   Energy pattern of acute grief reaction.

rebuild her life in a new way. We can note the lowered energy levels in all the centers and a general harmony of the interrelationships of the fields as there had not been time to develop adaptations or overcompensations.

When we see a similar pattern in a person who has not experienced a significant loss recently, we may justly begin to look for repressed grief. Often, the denial of mourning means that the individual never shed all the tears that needed to be released and the sadness is held as a constriction or block in the energy field. The person may feel it would be too overwhelming to bring the sadness to awareness and develops major constrictions in the energy field as time goes on. Depression is often a suppressed form of grief, a generalized adaptation, in which the individual is sad and functioning at half-mast most of the time.

Codependency and Childhood Abuse

Much has been written recently about personality patterns of individuals who grew up in dysfunctional families and later moved into distorted relationships in adulthood (Beattie, 1987; Black, 1982). It is not surprising, then, that these patterns can be seen in the energy field. The heart and sexual centers are usually wide open or overfilled with energy indicating the indiscriminate giving of love and affection even to unworthy parents or partners. The intuitive center, the brow chakra, is diminished or blocked so that the codependent cannot see with insight into others' motivations or realities.

Represented in figure 6.5 is the energetic description of a client who was constantly attracted to abusive men. Until evaluation of the energy field was done, she was not consciously aware of the abuse that occurred in early childhood. The energy pattern showed tremendous blocks in the pelvic area; holding in of the power center, the solar plexus; and signs of long-term imbalance in that every dimension of the field was affected. When this was brought to her attention in a safe and supportive environment, she began to recall, in short flashes, scenes of very early abuse that she could not comprehend or verbalize.

The lifetime impact of child abuse can be seen in the extreme distortions of the energy field. We are just beginning to comprehend the devastating effects of abuse that leave behind a

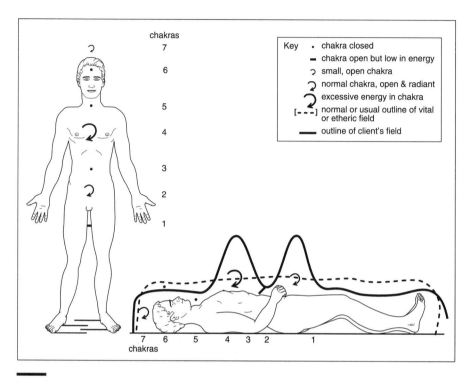

FIGURE 6.5   *Energy pattern associated with codependency and childhood abuse.*

legacy of distorted thinking and emotional patterns (Whitfield, 1987). We know it can take years to counteract these distortions through psychotherapy. From an energy-based point of view, we can assist the client in releasing old memories, which are literally blocks in the energy field, so that new thinking and feeling patterns can emerge. We will further explore the integration of psychotherapy and energy concepts in chapter 14.

Being Strong

In our culture denying feelings and being strong are highly valued. This thinking is further enhanced in the educational process of many health care professionals who are taught to be objective and impersonal at all times. Treating a patient as a diagnosis or an object to be moved from one technology to another preserves this kind of distancing. Unfortunately, the very qualities of human warmth and caring that could most help the patient are denied with this philosophy. Although holding in one's feelings may not cause active distress, it definitely blocks the flow of energy in the chakras and the field, creating a kind of invisible barrier that prevents the intuitive, creative potential and the capacity to enjoy life fully.

Many persons who have lived with these barriers in their energy fields experience vague symptoms of dissatisfaction. These may become more apparent in midlife when one begins asking, "Is this all there is?" Thus, what is often termed *midlife crisis* is another time to take stock of our human energy flows and to explore ways of opening safely to wider awareness, our sense of purpose, and meaning in life.

SUMMARY

We begin to note that energy field assessment could be valuable as a complement to traditional medical and psychological care. It is not enough to simply medicate or give talk-therapy. Use of energetic techniques to release blockages can speed the healing process for the client. This has rich implications for working with medical practitioners, body-oriented therapists, and psychotherapists. With a combination of appropriate energetic interventions and traditional practices, the client can move more quickly and effectively into personal change.

References

Bandler, R., & Grinder, J. (1982). *Reframing*. Moab, UT: Real People Press.

Beattie, M. (1987). *Codependent no more*. New York: Harper and Row.

Black, C. (1982). *It will never happen to me!* Denver: M.A.C. Printing and Publications Division.

Friedman, M., & Rosenmann, R. H. (1974). *Type A behavior and your heart*. Greenwich, CT: Fawcett Publishing.

Green, E., & Green, A. (1977). *Beyond biofeedback*. New York: Delta Books.

Karagulla, S., & Kunz, D. (1989). *The chakras and the human energy fields*. Wheaton, IL: Theosophical Publishing House.

Selye, H. (1978). *The stress of life*. New York: American Library.

Whitfield, C. L. (1987). *Healing the child within*. Deerfield Beach, FL: Health Communications, Inc.

3 HEALING TOUCH INTERVENTIONS

*T*hroughout recorded history many teachers and healers have described techniques of working with touch. The person who wishes to be a healer usually begins learning approaches to the client's energy field by studying with someone who is an expert. The techniques are often taught by word of mouth and handed down from one generation to the next rather than being written. In the healing interventions described in this part of the book, we have attempted to include available information about the most immediate source of each intervention, but this is by no means a complete history of its origin.

As skill in using techniques increases, healers may blend these practices into a personal style of working directly and intuitively with the client's energy. In the next five chapters we will explore specific techniques utilized in Healing Touch and discuss considerations for developing a practice of healing.

7 | THE BASIC TOOLS

Janet Mentgen, BSN, RN

Centering requires the exclusion of extraneous, distracting thoughts and feelings, focusing the attention on the immovable central core of being.

Benor, 1985

INTRODUCTION

In the health care field, the Krieger-Kunz method of Therapeutic Touch is the foremost and best-known energetic approach to healing work. Practiced under the guidelines published by the Nurse Healers — Professional Associates (1991), this 9-step technique is the currently recognized method of energy-based healing used in hospitals and nursing facilities across the United States.

THERAPEUTIC TOUCH

As a professor of nursing at New York University, Dr. Dolores Krieger introduced the concepts of Therapeutic Touch to her nursing students in 1972. Because of the innovative nature of the program, her students were called "Krieger's Krazies." The work has expanded since then and is taught at more than 80 major colleges and universities in this country and is known in more than

60 foreign countries through presentations and classes (Krieger, 1993, p. 5). Dr. Krieger describes Therapeutic Touch as "a contemporary interpretation of several ancient healing practices. These practices consist of learned skills for consciously directing or sensitively modulating human energies" (Krieger, 1993, p. 11).

The intervention of Therapeutic Touch is used to assist clients to repattern their energy in the direction of health and can be used alone or in conjunction with other modalities. The approach is useful for reducing pain and anxiety, promoting relaxation, and enhancing the body's natural restorative processes, as discussed in chapter 3 on research.

The organization that supports practitioners of Therapeutic Touch (TT), the Nurse Healers — Professional Associates, Inc., recommends the following guidelines:

- TT may be practiced by anyone who has successfully completed a beginning workshop which presents the theory and practice of TT.

- TT may be offered to anyone who could benefit from the technique.

- TT is an autonomous health care procedure performed within professional practice guidelines. (1991, p. 9)

Usually, 15 or 20 minutes is considered ample time for a TT treatment, and the practitioner adjusts the intervention to the needs of the client. In general, neonates, children, pregnant women, persons with psychiatric disorders, the elderly, and the acutely ill react more sensitively to the intervention.

PROCESSES OF THERAPEUTIC TOUCH

The following exercises will give you an opportunity to learn our understanding of the five most basic processes of Therapeutic Touch. They are (1) centering, (2) assessing the energy field, (3) smoothing or *unruffling* the field, (4) modulating or transferring energy, and (5) knowing when to stop. In subsequent chapters you will see ways you can use each process individually or integrate it into a longer healing session in conjunction with the other techniques that are described.

Sensing Energy

Sensing your own energy field is a good way to begin learning about energy. The steps described in the following exercise give you a way to practice increasing your sensitivity and to learn from your own experience. With practice, it can teach you much about your own energy field and enhance your sensitivity to energy. The exercise also requires focusing your attention by working with the breath, paying attention to the body, and refocusing whenever your attention wanders. Needless to say, this is not easy the first time, but it becomes much more natural with repetition and practice.

Essentially, you are learning how to bring the restless, sometimes wandering mind into calmer, more focused attention. We call this *centering*, and it is the basic tool for all energetic interventions whether for self-care or to assist others.

EXERCISE

Sensing Energy

1. Begin by taking several deep breaths, being careful to exhale completely, as if releasing air from a balloon. Blow out gently as if you were blowing out a candle. Sense the release of tension as you exhale, and connect with the joy of nature as you inhale.

2. Image bringing golden sunlight into your lungs as you inhale and releasing any darkness or heaviness as you exhale. Let the golden light flow to your heart, and, with the blood's circulation, image the flow of the light to each part of your body. Note where there is discomfort or a constriction in your body.

3. See the golden light flowing from the center of your chest to the shoulders, the arms, and the hands. Let the hands fill with the unlimited flow of this golden light and the quality of warmth and caring.

4. Maintaining your relaxed state, bring the palms of the hands opposite each other. Sense the fullness or warmth between them. Note how far you can separate the hands and still feel this fullness or warmth. Note how close together you can bring the hands without touching. Is there a difference? Explore the sensation, letting go of any goal or need to "do it right."

5. Continuing your work with gentle breaths to refocus when-ever your attention wanders, bring your awareness into the right index finger. Let the finger point at the left palm and draw a pattern at a distance of 1–3 inches as seen in figure 7.1. Note how this feels.

6. Bring your full attention into the left index finger and send your awareness into the right palm drawing another pattern. How does this feel? Is one hand more sensitive to sending or receiving than the other?

7. Gently bring your focus back to the palms of both hands. Let them play back and forth as you observe your experience. Simply let yourself enjoy the awareness and discovery from your own energies.

8. Bring the energized hands to rest on any part of the body that felt uncomfortable earlier. Continue to draw the golden light from the limitless universe into your body with the breath and your caring attention.

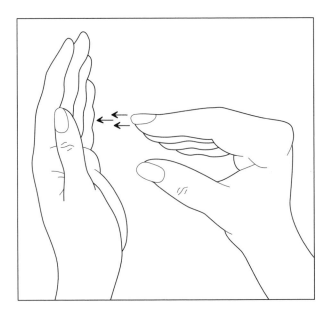

FIGURE 7.1 Sensing energy by directing index finger into opposite palm.

9. Gently release your focus and come back to the present making a note of what you have learned.

Centering

Practitioners of Therapeutic Touch, Healing Touch, and other energy-oriented modalities find that centering and working with inner awareness is the most vital part of their work. If we are centered, we can move with confidence and a full, flowing, protective energy field into difficult situations. If we are off-center and discombobulated, we stumble around, becoming more and more frazzled with less and less to give. Energetically speaking, centering brings us into harmony with the Universal Energy Flow. Even without specific knowledge of energies, others can sense the difference when we are in a state of balance.

The exercise for centering is specifically designed to help you learn to develop your inner focus and later learn to do it quickly in clinical settings. With practice, this kind of daily centering gives you a delightful way to begin or end the day or to calm yourself during a break in the work schedule. It is a good idea to practice every day for 15 minutes until it becomes a natural part of your daily routine, like brushing your teeth. More rapid centering, at a patient's beside for instance, is possible after the longer method becomes automatic. With practice, just taking an intentional breath and imaging the peaceful place is enough to connect you with the centered state. With frequent repetition, centering and focusing can happen quickly whenever needed. You may even find that you are walking in and out of the centered state most of the time and that your work flows more easily as a result.

EXERCISE

Centering

1. Working with the breath, release any heaviness, the accumulated debris of the day, worry, or concerns as you exhale. Do this three times, then ease into a very comfortable position.

2. In your mind's eye, allow yourself to go to a time when you felt very peaceful in nature. This may be a place you have visited or a picture you remember. Seat yourself comfortably and just allow yourself to enjoy the immediate moment of being in this peaceful place.

3. See the colors around you. Notice the lighting, the shadows, the shadings of the colors. Notice the textures around you — smooth, rough, rocky, flowing. Notice clouds and other beauty. Let your awareness of this lovely place grow.

4. Let yourself hear the sounds — a bird in the distance, the sound of flowing water, the rustle of leaves as a gentle breeze blows by.

5. Feel the breeze on your cheeks and sense the cooling. Sense the warmth of the sun. Feel the relaxation of this peaceful place inside your body. Feel the relaxation in any areas of tension or stress.

6. Smell the flavors of this peaceful place — the leaves on the forest floor or the fresh salt air of the sea. Enjoy all the senses as you take the inner journey to this peaceful place.

7. Gently let your awareness shift back to the present time taking with you the feeling of relaxation and peacefulness. Know you can return to this experience whenever you choose.

Assessment of the Energy Field

After centering, you are ready to practice sensing another person's energy field. Assessment is a step that allows you to sense another's field without judgment or preconceived notions. The following exercise will help you to develop skills in assessing your client's energy field.

EXERCISE

Assessing the Energy Field

1. To begin, have a friend or interested person sit comfortably in a chair while you stand behind.

2. Using both hands, scan above the head 1–6 inches away from the body. Sense the energy field around the head, neck, and shoulders paying attention to what your hands sense. Does the energy feel cool, warm, bumpy, smooth, or tingly? Is there a sensation of fullness, vibration, pulsation, or depletion? Do you feel pulled in or pushed away? Which parts feel the same, and where are things different?

3. Share with your friend what you noticed and ask if this has any meaning for her. If you are working with a group, it is helpful to assess another person's field in the same manner, noting how the fields of two people are similar or different.

4. Hold your hands above the crown chakra, or the fontanel area, to discover if it feels warmer or cooler than the neck and shoulders. Hold your hands out as far as you can reach on both sides of the head and find the edge of the energy field. This edge or outer layer may extend farther than you can reach with your hands. Have your friend help you by reporting when she feels your hands in her field. Note if the field is symmetrical on both sides or distorted in some way.

5. Work your way all around your friend's body, 1–6 inches away, noting areas of difference. The energy is smooth and symmetrical in a balanced energy field, so any differences are clues to areas of imbalance and disruption. Scan the back of the head, neck, and shoulders, following with the front of the face and neck. Standing to one side of the body, scan the chest and abdomen, then assess down the arm to the hands and down the leg to the foot. Move to the other side and repeat the assessment. From the front of the body, scan over the chest, abdomen, thighs, and calves, ending with the tops of the feet. Finally, assess the back, scanning both sides and the spine.

6. Share the differences you noted with your friend and find out what meaning these findings have for her.

Discussion   It is always best to be very neutral about information you sense, letting the awareness of any meaning come from the client. There is a world of difference between saying, "I noticed some heat over the right shoulder area" and interpreting, "You have heat and congestion here that must come from too much exercise."

Sometimes the client makes no conscious connection between what you sensed and any current symptoms. This does not mean you were inaccurate. Remember that problems appear to manifest first in the energy field before becoming identifiable physical symptoms. A pervading denial of the physical body exists in our culture, so people are often not even aware of discomfort until it is acute and above their pain thresholds. Many times people have come to us after an assessment and recalled some stress on the previous day or a prior injury that they had forgotten about.

Development of assessment skills requires frequent practice. Try sensing the energy of at least 20 people and notice the variations among them. Feel the head of someone who has an active headache and you will learn what this condition does to the energy field. Comparisons help you to learn differences. Is there a difference between tension, sinus, or migraine headaches? How does pain, acute and chronic, feel? Practice scanning both healthy and ill persons to help develop your sensitivity. Remembering to center first will, of course, greatly help you to increase your sensory acuity.

Unruffling or Smoothing the Field

Unruffling, using calm and rhythmic hand movements to clear the energy field of a *ruffled* or congested area, is one of the basic healing techniques described by Dr. Dolores Krieger (1993, p. 65). Unruffling may be used by itself as a simple, effective technique in any setting or in conjuction with the modulation of energy described in the next section. Unruffling requires the focused intention of the healer and allows for gradual relaxation of the healee through relief of pain, discomfort, or anxiety. Both hands are placed 1–6 inches above the client's skin in the etheric layer of the energy field. The hands are held open with the flat surface of the palm brushing down and away from above to below the problem site.

The client can be in a sitting position or lying down while the healer's hands move in the etheric layer, down and away from the body, utilizing either short or long connected strokes in a graceful, sweeping motion. Figure 7.2 shows unruffling in action, and the following exercise gives further detail.

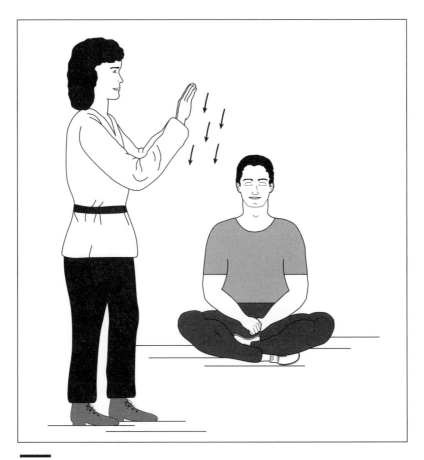

FIGURE 7.2   Unruffling or smoothing the energy field.

When used immediately after a traumatic injury, unruffling seems to reconnect the damaged tissue and assist the return of a normal flow of energy within the body. When unruffling, be sure to move the hands completely off the body far enough for the blockage, pain, or discomfort to drop away. This motion may be exaggerated as needed, especially if the energy or pain feels stuck. The purpose is to unlock the stagnated energy and to reestablish the flow in the affected body part. Unruffling may be done over a specific part of the energy field or over the entire body. In emotional depression, unruffling very often helps shift the feeling state of the patient to a more positive sense of self.

EXERCISE

Unruffling

1. Select an area that is in need of smoothing or balancing from your assessment of another's energy field. (You may also ask your client or friend which physical area most needs assistance.)

2. After centering yourself, brush away the congested area just above the skin by repeatedly sweeping with the hands from above the site to below the site.

3. Do this for about 3 to 5 minutes noting changes in the field. Have your partner describe any sensations and share any perceptions. Look for changes in skin color, temperature, voice level, respiration, and pulse rate that come with the relaxation response and activation of the parasympathetic nervous system (Benson, 1987).

Transfer or Modulation of Energy

Direct laying on of hands for the modulation of the client's energy is the second basic healing technique described by Krieger (1993, pp. 70–71) and by Alice Bailey (1978, p. 649). The hands are placed directly on the selected area of the body and held still to allow a transfer or modulation of energy from the healer to the healee. This seems to allow the client's energy to move toward balance.

The goal is to bring balance and harmony to the areas of the field that have been blocked or congested. The technique involves simply resting the hands on the specific area of the body and holding them in place for a period of time, usually 3 to 5 minutes. The hands may be kept in place until the healer feels a change, such as fullness or warmth, which is a clue the energy has shifted.

The clues of energy change are subtle: an area that was blocked and cool becomes warm; a hot area cools down; pulsation may begin; throbbing may stop; or pain may intensify, release, and quietly subside. There may be vibration, tingling, quieting, or other sensations. The healer needs to observe when change has occurred and when the specific area being treated begins to feel as symmetrical and smooth as the rest of the body.

EXERCISE

Modulating or Transferring Energy

1. With your hand scan, identify an area of the client's body that is in need of balancing, or ask your client where direct touch would be helpful.

2. After centering, place your hands directly on the identified area that has energy disturbance or pain. To work more deeply in the tissues, place the hands on opposite sides of the body.

3. Hold the hands in this position for 3 to 5 minutes noting any shifts in the energy or pulsation, and listen to feedback from the client. Your hands act as the focal point of your attention and allow the client's energy to modulate itself toward balance beneath them.

Closure

You may wish to reassess the field after either unruffling or modulating energy and repeat either of these processes if further balancing is needed. Recognizing when it is time to stop is the final step. Closure is indicated when there are no longer any perceivable differences in the energy field and when there is a sense of balance and symmetry. Usually, there are also shifts in the client's affect, as well as deeper breathing, a flush of the skin, or other signs of relaxation that let you know when you have finished.

The client should have time to rest quietly, letting the changes in the energy field integrate throughout its layers. There is often a feeling of calmness and peacefulness. Let the client rest as long as possible; in hospital settings, the patient may drift into sleep that offers a good time for undisturbed rest. If the client needs to go back to work or drive somewhere, it is helpful to talk about the experience as a way of stimulating alertness and making sure the client is in full consciousness.

Documentation   It is also valuable to document the results of the intervention, citing what the symptoms were, the procedure used, objective and subjective observations, and feedback from the client. In addition, notice any effects of the intervention in you as the helping person, as energetic interventions can effect changes, emotionally and physically, in the healer as well.

SUMMARY

We have described the five essential elements of Therapeutic Touch — centering, assessment, unruffling, transferring or modulating energy, and closure. Combined, they constitute an entire Therapeutic Touch sequence of 15 to 20 minutes and usually yield the effects that have been described in the extensive research literature. Each technique can also be used by itself, provided the healer is centered and intentional. Each process can also be used in conjunction with the other systemic and localized techniques that will be described in subsequent chapters.

References

Bailey, A. (1978). *Esoteric healing* (p. 649). New York: Lucis Publishing Co.

Benor, D. (1985, March). Believe it and you'll be it. *Psi Research,* pp. 42–43.

Benson, H. (1987). *Your maximum mind.* New York: Random House.

Krieger, D. (1993). *Accepting your power to heal.* Santa Fe, NM: Bear and Co.

Nurse Healers — Professional Associates, Inc. (1991). Therapeutic Touch policy and procedure for health professionals. *The Cooperative Connection, III:*9.

8 | FULL BODY TECHNIQUES

Janet Mentgen, BSN, RN

We are not interested in developing psychonoetic powers for their own sake, for the purpose of creating phenomena. We want to develop such powers only for purposes of healing, to be of service to our fellow human beings.

Daskalos as quoted in Markides, 1987

INTRODUCTION

As the name implies, full body techniques are used on the entire body, to complete balancing of the entire energy field. Although they usually take longer to complete than a single intervention, they have a more sustained effect. The healer uses a full body technique when there is a systemic or chronic disease process affecting the entire body. Specifically, these techniques can be utilized for toxicity, trauma, anxiety, or other systemic imbalance. A full body technique is preferred whenever there is enough time because of the greater effect on the entire field.

FULL BODY TECHNIQUES

Full Body Connection

The Full Body Connection has been developed from a variety of sources and is a basic technique used in the Healing Touch

Program. This technique combines the concepts of the Chakra Connection (Joy, 1979) and Chelation as taught by Rosalyn Bruyere (1989) and Barbara Brennan (1987).

To *chelate* means to claw out or to spin out. The technique is done with a spinning motion of your energy, throwing the auric debris in the energy field to the edges with a centrifuge-like motion. It is a much more focused directing of energy than the gentle holding done with Therapeutic Touch. This directing of your focus is necessary to override the current energy blockage due to congestion and constriction in the client's energy field.

Technique   During this technique the client is usually lying on his back, although it can be modified to accommodate someone lying on the stomach or side or sitting in a chair. The steps of this technique are illustrated and described in the Full Body Connection exercise.

Each of the points in the technique are held from 1 to 3 minutes depending on the degree of healing and energizing work that needs to be done or on the time available. The healer stands on the right side of the patient when performing this technique. Move the lower hand to the upper hand position first in order to maintain contact with the person at all times.

Effect   The Full Body Connection can be used by itself or as a preparation for further intervention work. The procedure can also indicate energy blocks when you note that some areas of the body are less responsive than others. For instance, rotations may occur at different speeds, and temperatures over a chakra area may differ. By balancing the client with the Full Body Connection, other specific interventions can be added readily and are usually even more effective.

EXERCISE

Full Body Connection[1]

1. After centering, begin by holding the sole of the right foot and the right ankle, holding until a flow occurs between your palms. You may feel movement or spinning in your own body

------

[1] Figures reprinted with permission from Janet L. Mentgen, Program Administrator, Healing Touch.

or hands as part of the chelation. Spin the energy flow clockwise to clear this area of any congestion, fast enough to rotate the energy to the point of release. Do this until the area underneath your hands feels full, balanced, and free, or until you cannot get any further movement.

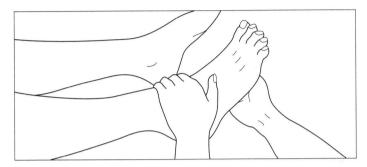

2. Move the hands to the right ankle and knee while chelating, or spinning, your own body with a clockwise rotation.

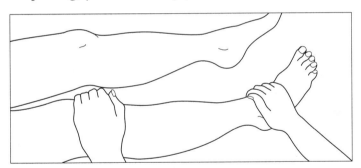

3. Move to connect the right knee and the right hip joint.

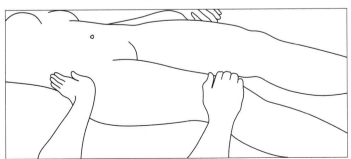

4. Reach across the body and hold between the palms of your hands the sole of the left foot and the left ankle.

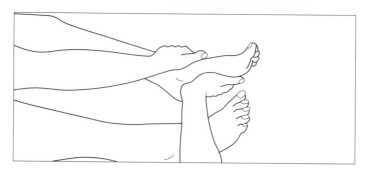

5. Move to the left ankle and knee.

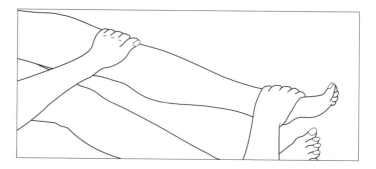

6. Hold the left knee and hip joint.

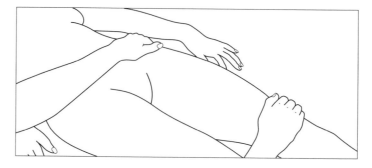

7. Hold both hip joints. At this time you may check the right and left sides of the body for balance as you sense the energy flow through the hips.

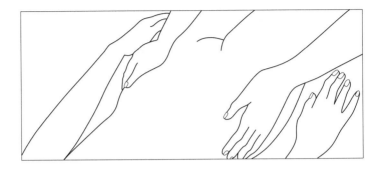

8. Place the right hand at the root chakra, between the legs about 6 inches below the floor of the perineum, or above the pubic bone, and the left hand on the sacral chakra, slightly below the umbilicus. Chelate these two chakras by spinning in a clockwise direction until they match, balance, and feel equal. The best way to spin the root chakra is for the healer to spin her own root chakra with a clockwise rotation and let the healee's chakra match the spin.

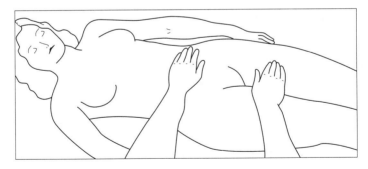

9. Slide the lower right hand underneath the upper left hand at the sacral chakra, pause with the doubled hands for a few seconds, and then move the left or upper hand to the solar plexus center. Spin the centers clockwise in a downward spiral, matching the levels of depth between your hands.

Continue to spin clockwise until the energy feels smooth and even, or until you are aware that you have held it long enough.

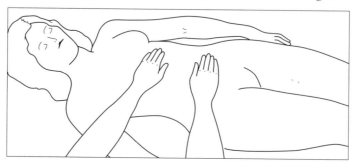

10. Keeping the left hand on the solar plexus move the right or lower hand to the spleen area on the left side of the body over the lower edge of the rib cage. Then move the left hand to the right side of the body over the liver area and spin clockwise again. Hold until there is a sense of smooth flowing and balance.

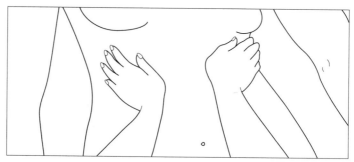

11. Move your right hand back to the solar plexus and your left or upper hand to the heart center area. Feel the hands spin downward in the spiral to match the two centers, then chelate your own body clockwise.

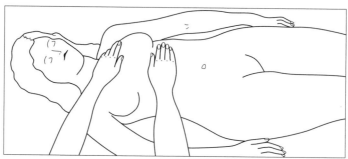

12. Using your right hand take the client's right hand and lock thumbs matching your palms together and put your left hand on the wrist. Send the energy through your palms creating a flow and continue balancing.

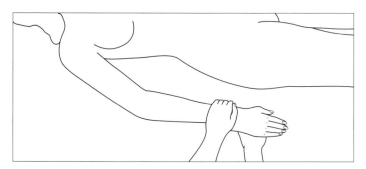

13. Move your hands upward to the right wrist and elbow, continuing your own chelation motion.

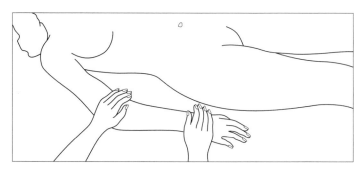

14. Hold the elbow and shoulder.

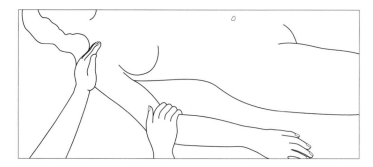

15. Reach across the body to hold the left palm and wrist.

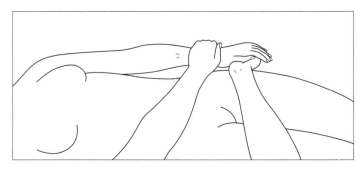

16. Hold the left wrist and elbow.

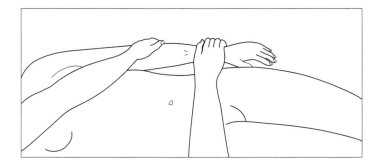

17. Hold the left elbow and shoulder.

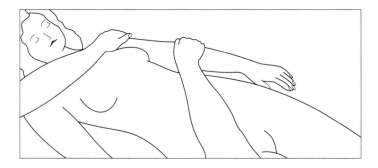

18. Hold both shoulders, again checking the right and left sides for balance, and chelate this area.

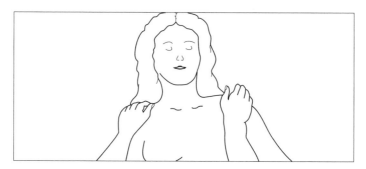

19. Return the right hand to the heart center and the left hand to the throat. The hand is held lightly over the notch of the neck between the collar bones. (An alternate position is to hold behind the neck with the left hand.)

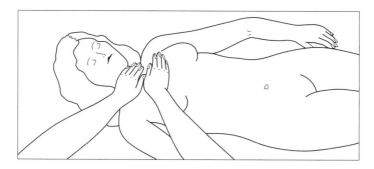

20. Bring the left hand to the brow center and move the right hand to the front of the throat.

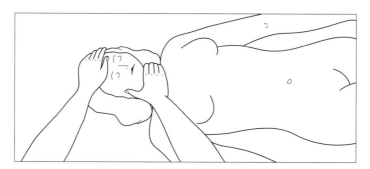

21. Place the left hand on the top of the head at the crown center with the right hand on the brow.

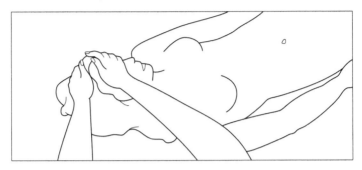

22. The process is completed by holding the crown with the right hand and extending the left hand straight above the crown with the palm pointed outward toward the transpersonal point that extends about 18 inches above the head.

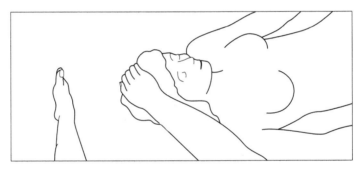

Etheric Vitality

Etheric Vitality is a technique described by a Greek healer as a preparatory meditation for the caregiver (Markides, 1987, pp. 58–60). Labeled by Janet Mentgen, Etheric Vitality is a self-directed meditation to prepare the helper and client for relaxation and centering. This technique opens the chakra system in the healee, who may describe feeling a variety of body sensations.

Doing this meditation with the hands on the client's head is a preparation for healing interventions that follow. It is a powerful centering process as it opens the channel for connecting with the Universal Energy Flow of the healee as well as the healer.

EXERCISE

Etheric Vitality

1. Sit or stand at the head of the table. The healee should be lying supine with a pillow underneath the knees, keeping the back straight and the head flat. (This can also be done with the healee sitting in a chair and the healer standing behind the chair.)

2. Place the palms of your hands on the crown center of the client's head and hold this position for 7 to 10 minutes, or you may hold your hands in the field above the head. Feel the energy flow, sensing when the body is fully open energetically and when it is time to stop.

3. With your eyes closed or opened, repeat silently to yourself, "I focus all my attention on the soles of my feet, nothing else but the soles of the feet. My entire attention is on the soles of my feet. I hold my full attention on the soles of my feet."

4. Continuing the silent meditation, say, "Now I move the energy upward. I feel the movement to the ankles. I am aware of only the soles of my feet and my ankles, nothing else. I hold my attention on my ankles and feet."

5. "Now I move the energy upward from my ankles to my knees. I feel the energy moving upward as I inhale and become aware of my knees, ankles, and feet. I hold in my awareness only the feeling of my knees, ankles, and feet. Nothing else enters my mind."

6. "I again breathe the energy from the knees into the hips and feel the energy move into the hips and pelvis. I focus my attention on my legs, hips, and pelvis. Now I breathe the light energy outward and surround my entire legs in glowing white light. I feel the healing white light all around both legs and my pelvis."

7. "I now breathe the energy into the abdomen and imagine a nebula of blue-white light swirling clockwise. I focus entirely on the nebula of blue-white light rotating clockwise in my abdomen."

8. "I breathe the energy into my heart and imagine a nebula of rose-white light, swirling clockwise in my heart. I focus entirely on the nebula of rose-white light watching as it swirls within my heart."

9. "I breathe the energy into my throat and imagine a nebula of orange-white light within my throat area. I watch intensely the nebula of orange-white light within my throat as it swirls clockwise. Then I watch this nebula of intense light separate and move to each shoulder then down my arms into my palms, activating my healing hands to do the work I am about to do. I imagine the white light surrounding my arms and expanding outward all around my arms and hands."

10. "I breathe the light into my head and imagine a nebula of gold-white light inside my head and expanding outward, surrounding my head until a shimmering gold-white light is all around my head and around my entire body. I remain in this shimmering goldwhite light as I do the healing work."

Magnetic Unruffle

Magnetic Unruffling is a technique that was developed and identified by Janet Mentgen for the purpose of clearing the entire body of congested energy. It is used when there is a history of long-term prescription or recreational drug use, after anesthesia, chronic pain, trauma, breathing of polluted air, environmental sensitivities, smoking (even when the person has not smoked for a number of years), and for systemic disease. This technique cleanses the body's energy field in a systemic way. It also assists in releasing emotional debris and unresolved feelings, such as anger, fear, worry, tension, and anxiety.

Sometimes the energy will clear in the upper portion of the body and become denser in the legs and lower body. Completing each sweep from head to toe without interruption is important for this reason. Stopping to work in one area would impede the flow that cleanses the field. The goal of the Magnetic Unruffle is to completely clear the entire energy field of any accumulations or constrictions.

EXERCISE

Magnetic Unruffle

1. The healee lies on the table, on his back with shoes, belt, and glasses removed and clothing comfortably loose. The healer begins by placing the hands about 12 inches above the healee's head. The fingers are spread, relaxed, and curled, and the thumbs are either touching each other or close together. Use a long continuous raking motion over the entire body starting above the head and moving down the center of the body to the feet. The movement of the hands from head to toe should be in one smooth, continuous motion, uninterrupted until coming off the body beyond the toes. Continue the pull beyond the body until the sensation of energy drops away. The movement should take about 30 seconds from head to toe, going slowly enough to feel energy gather in your hands.

2. Repeat this motion from the head to beyond the feet about 30 times, or for about 15 minutes, until the energy feels smooth and even, like glass, over the entire body. Alternatives are to do one side first and then move to the other, or to turn the client over and do the same process on the back. Your hands may perceive a tremendous buildup of dense energy as you unruffle the energy field. A useful metaphor is to imagine the hands as magnets and the debris in the energy field like iron filings that are attracted to the magnet and stick to it. Each time your hands come off the body you will need to shake or pull off the sensation of the iron filings on your hands.

3. Each stroke may feel different as new layers of the energy field are reached. Visualize the layers of the field as the growth rings within a tree. Each year a new ring of the tree is created and is stored in the structure of the trunk; in a similar way, the body creates new energy layers, one by one, as we grow and change. A buildup of congested energy can occur, which may contain old memories, pain, or traumatic events. As each layer is released, the next layer emerges.

Chakra Spread

The Chakra Spread was demonstrated to the author by Catherine Fanslow (1988). The process described in the Chakra Spread exercise is used in hospice care for the terminally ill or for persons in severe pain. Families who are sitting with a dying patient can also benefit from this technique to reduce their own stress levels.

The many applications of this technique include severe pain, before and after medical procedures, pre- and postsurgery intervention, severe stress reactions, to ease any critical life transition, and to assist someone who is choosing to enter a profound meditation. This powerful technique takes a person to a deeper level of healing than is achieved by most techniques, so its use should be reserved for special needs and sacred moments in healing.

Technique   Usually, the healer lies on his back on a massage table or a bed. The hand-holding position is very comforting for the anxious or dying person. Even if the client is unable to speak, awareness of others' presence and comfort is still experienced. It is also helpful to show family or friends sitting at the bedside how to hold the hand of a loved one in the locked thumb position with the other hand on top, assisting them to offer the gift of touch. A quiet environment, subdued lighting, slow relaxing music of a meditative nature or baroque classical music assist the process. The healee may have special requests for music.

All of your movements in this technique need to be very slow and gentle, avoiding any jarring or sudden, quick movements. Remember that the patient may be very weak, severely traumatized, hypersensitive, or extremely sedated. Any sudden movement may intensify the pain or disrupt the body's energy field.

With this process, pain will often diminish, or the client may relax deeply and fall asleep. After the person has relaxed completely, fears and other emotional issues that need to be processed will sometimes surface. The healer or family members need to be available for this sharing.

The technique can also be done in silence and takes only about 10 to 15 minutes. It is better to repeat the technique frequently than to extend the time. Family members or caregivers can learn the procedure so relief may be offered whenever they are present. All caregivers need to do the Chakra Spread in a similar manner as familiarity and repetition provide comfort when the client is in a terminal, comatose, or unconscious state.

As a variation, the Chakra Spread may also be completed in a chair. Security is necessary because the patient may relax, fall asleep, and slip out of the chair. Begin by holding the feet and the hands. Then, go behind the chair and begin to spread gently and slowly three times at the top of the head, the crown, brow, throat, and heart centers. Move to the front of the healee and squat or kneel to spread the chakras at the solar plexus, abdomen, root, hips, knees, and ankles. Pull the energy off the tops of the feet. Repeat the sequence three times and end by holding one hand while placing the other hand on the heart.

EXERCISE

Chakra Spread

1. Begin by holding the sole of the foot with the palm of your hand and place the other hand on top of the foot or ankle. Hold for at least a minute to open the energy center at the sole of the foot as a release for pain, tension, or anxiety. Hold the other foot in like manner for a minute.

2. Go to one side of the patient and hold the hand by locking thumbs, with your palm touching the client's palm and placing your other hand on the back of the patient's hand. Hold for at least a minute to open the energy flow in the palm chakra, creating a drain or release for accumulated stress. Repeat this hold on the other hand.

3. Move to the top of the head and bring both hands together into the energy field above the crown chakra. You will feel the edges of the chakra as you enter the field. Gently and slowly spread both hands outward as far as you can reach. Repeat this three times, noting changes in the energy field.

4. Spread each lower chakra in similar fashion in the following order: crown, brow, throat, heart, solar plexus, abdomen, and root chakra. Notice how each chakra area feels. Continue by spreading the energy areas around the knees and the ankles.

5. Pull the energy off each foot by placing one hand above the foot and one hand below the sole of the foot. The pulling away resembles bringing a column of light off the foot.

6. Return to the crown and repeat the spread on each chakra three more times.

7. Repeat this sequence one more time, completing three entire rounds.

8. To complete the technique, return to one hand of your client and hold it again in the locked thumb position while placing your other hand on the heart center area of the patient.

Etheric Unruffle

In 1991, Rod Campbell, an Australian healer, demonstrated a technique to Janet Mentgen. She modified it and labeled the procedure Etheric Unruffling. This very simple procedure creates a profound effect by working on the etheric or vital level, which is closest to the skin in the interface between the physical body and emotional layer.

Technique   The healer usually sits next to the client who is lying on a bed or table. Place the hands slightly above the body and gently move the hands until you begin to feel the etheric field. Where there is disturbance or a problem you will feel a difference in the field from the smooth flow of a clear field to the turbulence or vibration of a blocked area. Work this area by moving the hands in any direction following the energetic pathways. It may feel as if you are combing the field, untangling strands, or repairing a chakra.

Etheric Unruffle teaches the healer to trust the energy as a guide. Release any personal attachment to predicted outcomes, other techniques, or expectations, and simply follow the energy. Let the energy speak for itself. Follow the energy by moving the hands in the client's field for an extended period of time, noting the condition and problems you encounter in the field. Advanced Healing Touch practitioners have done this technique for longer periods of time, up to an hour, in congested or complicated fields to release energy blockage.

This is the simplest of all the techniques described. However, the development of the healer must be sufficient to understand and read the energetic response in order for this to be effective. The process is done until the energy field feels clear and smooth. It is essential that the healer be mature, centered, and very attuned intuitively to the client's field.

SUMMARY

All full body techniques have an effect on the physical as well as other layers of the energy field. The initial effect of relaxation is sometimes followed by other forms of release, such as decreased pain perception, increased mental acuity, or emotional catharsis. The increased sense of well-being may last for several days or weeks depending on the responsiveness of the client's energy system.

References

Brennan, B. (1987). *Hands of light* (pp. 201–233). New York: Bantam Books.

Bruyere, R. (1989, October). Workshop on energetic healing. Glendale, CA: Healing Light Center Church.

Fanslow, C. (1988, October). Nurse Healers — Professional Associates Conference. Wichita, KS.

Joy, B. (1979). *Joy's way* (pp. 271–275). Los Angeles: J. P. Tarcher, Inc.

Markides, K. (1987). *Homage to the sun* (p. 8). New York: Arkana Books, Penguin Group.

9 LOCALIZED AND SPECIFIC TECHNIQUES

Janet Mentgen, BSN, RN

Thank you, my friend,
For you have shared your pain.
Now we can work together
As we surrender to the Powers
Beyond ourselves in seeking release
From the twisted turbulence
Within.

Hover-Kramer, 1993

INTRODUCTION

Specific techniques may be selected by the caregiver to accomplish specific healing outcomes. Having adequate time during an interaction with a client to find the most effective treatment is sometimes a challenge, especially in clinical settings. These guidelines are designed to help the healer select the appropriate technique quickly and to expedite the treatment of localized conditions.

SPECIFIC TECHNIQUES

Ultrasound

The technique of Ultrasound penetrates deeply into the body. Deep tissue penetration is effective for pain in arthritic joints, for stopping internal bleeding, for sealing lacerations, and for work around the eyes or ears. Ultrasound can be effective for fractured bones, tendonitis, joint injuries, and tumors. It can be used anywhere on the body where a deeply penetrating intervention is needed.

Ultrasound is always available because it requires only your hands and knowledge. If we were shipwrecked on a deserted island, we could use this energetic form of Ultrasound. As one of the first aid techniques of the future, Ultrasound is effective on all occasions where immediate relief from trauma is needed, establishing the process of self-healing to repair damaged tissue. The distressed pattern is broken up and reorganization of energy can occur quickly with the use of the energetic tool formed by the hand (see figure 9.1).

Animals especially respond to Ultrasound with immediate wound repair. Large gaping wounds woven together with

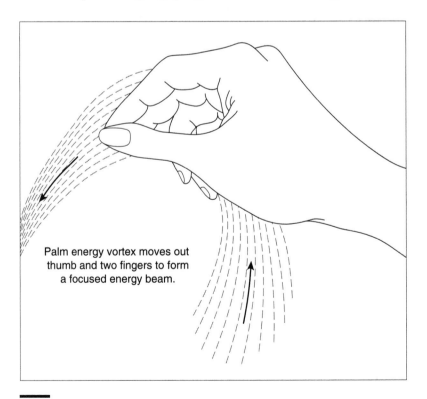

Palm energy vortex moves out thumb and two fingers to form a focused energy beam.

FIGURE 9.1　Ultrasound.

Ultrasound will often shrink to a tiny scab by the next morning. Experiment to see how quickly this technique assists healing. Most Healing Touch practitioners find that repeated work with Ultrasound is even more effective than a single application.

EXERCISE

Ultrasound

1. This technique is done by holding the thumb and first and second fingers together, directing energy from the palm chakra out the fingers and thumb. Imagine a beam of light coming from the fingers and thumb that is directed into the client's body.

2. Place the opposite hand behind the body part on which you are working. You can sense the beam of the light's deep penetration by feeling it in the palm of the opposing hand.

3. Try this on someone's wrist by putting one hand underneath the wrist and sending energy through the fingers and thumb of the other hand on top of the wrist.

4. To use Ultrasound, move the whole hand in any direction desired with the fingers pointed toward the area for about 3 to 5 minutes. Keep moving the hand continuously while doing Ultrasound, just as a physical therapist would move a mechanical ultrasound head.

Laser

The Laser technique is very similar to Ultrasound. This time, one or more fingers are held still and pointed toward the problem area with the sensation of an intermittent pulsing light penetrating deeply into the tissue. Laser can be effective with isolated pain such as a toothache, TMJ (temporal mandibular joint) problems, or any situation where spot healing is needed.

The Laser can be used for cutting, sealing, and breaking up congestion. It is sometimes used with just one finger pointed directly toward the body. An alternative is to use all the fingers pointed toward each other on opposite sides of the body to intensify the intersection of energy flows and to activate a specific area within the body. The Laser appears to be very powerful and is used for only a few seconds or up to a minute.

Mind Clearing

Mind Clearing is a technique taught by Rudy Noel, who studied extensively with Rosalyn Bruyere. Mind Clearing is used for relaxation and to focus the mind. It has become a favorite technique of Healing Touch students over the years. Family members can be taught this technique, and it is ideal for sharing in a relationship because it cannot be done easily on oneself.

Technique   For Mind Clearing the client is lying on his back, away from the headboard of a bed so the head can be reached easily. The healer may be standing or sitting. This technique can also be done while the client is lying on the floor or on a massage table with the healer sitting at the client's head. Another option is for the client simply to sit on a chair with the healer standing behind. However, the best results come when the client is lying down, due to the profound relaxation induced. Hold each of the steps illustrated and described in the following exercise for 1 to 3 minutes.

The client may drift to sleep or be fully relaxed. Process any thoughts or feelings that arose during the interaction. The client may share deeper levels of awareness after the body has had an opportunity to relax in this profound way, so plan some time for this exchange.

An alternate way to do the Mind Clearing is to use the palms of the hands instead of the fingertips. The effect of this is more soothing with less deep penetration into the tissues. As before, each hold is from 1 to 3 minutes.

EXERCISE

Mind Clearing[1]

1. After centering, begin by holding the fingers lightly just above the collar bone on each side of the throat. This establishes

------

[1] Mind Clearing sequence reprinted with permission from Rev. Rudy Noel, CET.

attunement between healer and healee and begins the flow of energy.

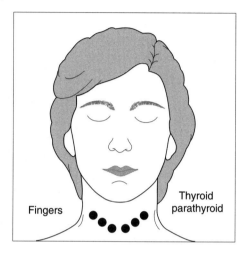

2. Put one hand on the center of the back of the head where the skull meets the neck. Find the notch in the occipital ridge and place the middle finger in the notch. Two fingers of the opposite hand rest between the eyebrows in the middle of the forehead.

Notice that the middle fingers will be pointing toward each other, intersecting through the midbrain. The touch is featherlight, so gentle there will be no mark of pressure left on the forehead.

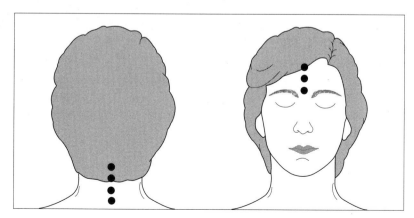

3. Place both hands under the head and wrap the fingers around the occipital ridge. Then lift the head gently with light pressure under the ridge (this usually feels good to the client). Pull the neck toward you, putting slight tension on the muscles of the neck. You may wish to ask the client if more or less pressure is needed.

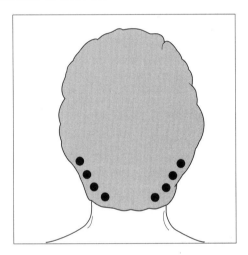

4. Hold the fingers of both hands around the skull like a cap with the thumbs on the crown of the head in the fontanel area. This point on top of the head affects blood pressure, and this hold can be used to reduce hypertension.

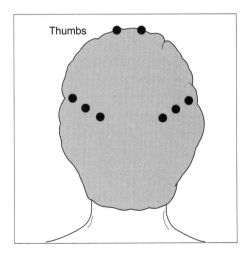

5. Balance the right and left hemispheres of the brain by placing the middle finger of each hand on a point above and slightly behind the ear at the hairline where you can feel a pulse. The pulse may feel uneven on each side at first, but with holding the pulses will move to a smooth, more balanced rhythm.

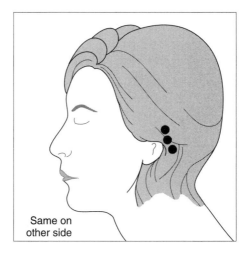

Same on other side

6. Set three fingers of each hand on a line from the inside of the eyebrows to the hairline, forming a **V**. Your elbows will be flared out and away from your body.

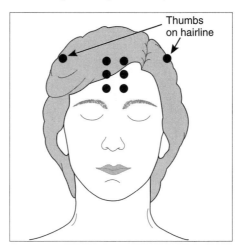

Thumbs on hairline

7. Spread the fingers to form a wider V to the outside of the eyebrow. This opens the window to the intuitive center sometimes called the third eye, and will be the peak of relaxation in the technique. The client will often experience images, dreams, colors, or deep sleep.

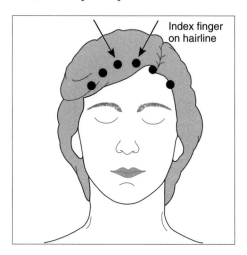

Index finger on hairline

8. Have the client open the mouth or yawn to help you find the mandibular joint. Then, have him close the mouth and massage this joint in the energy field by rotating your fingers using a circular motion.

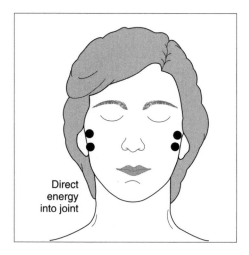

Direct energy into joint

9. Stroke three times from the middle of the brow, across the forehead, and down the cheeks over the mandibular joint. Add any additional gentle massage to the face and ears that seems appropriate.

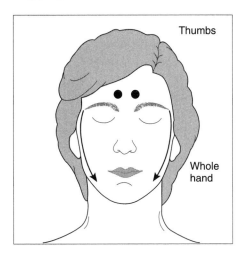

10. Softly brush the cheeks with the palms, and cup the hands lightly around the jaw so the fingers point to the throat.

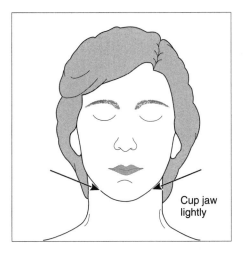

11. Finish with a gentle kiss, a light touch to the forehead, or a gesture, such as squeezing the shoulders, that lets the person know you are finished.

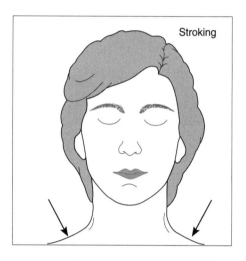

Magnetic Pain Drain

The Magnetic Pain Drain is a useful technique for acute and painful areas as it helps to remove pain or congestion in the energy field. As in other energy-based techniques, the healer is centered, still, and attuned to that which is for the highest good of the client. The basic concept in the technique is to use the left hand as the receiver of energy and the right hand as the release or sender of energetic material. Usually, the client will relax deeply and report relief of discomfort in 3 to 5 minutes with each of the two positions described in the following exercise.

EXERCISE

Magnetic Pain Drain

1. Place the left hand on the area that hurts or feels congested, and hold the right hand downward and away from the body. This siphons the energy from the client's body and out the healer's right hand. The healer may sometimes feel the activity move through her body. Usually, the energy will travel into the healer's left hand, up the arm, across the shoulders to the right arm, and leave the body through the hand. A pumping action with the right hand will speed up the process. Hold this position until the movement or sensation of pulling through stops and you are completely free of any pressure.

2. Reverse the hands, placing the right hand on the client's problem area and holding the left hand upward to bring in the healing energy from the Universal Energy Field. This allows the void that occurred from the draining action to fill with light and warmth. Remember that any energy drained off is neutral, does not have a negative or positive quality, and quickly dissipates into the Universal Energy Field.

Spiral Meditation

The Spiral Meditation is fully described in *Joy's Way* (Joy, 1979) and can be utilized as a meditation to open the energy field at the beginning of a healing sequence. It is also effective as a technique for opening energy centers that are blocked or constricted in energy flow. Because of its focus on the heart center, the Spiral Meditation is also effective in strengthening the heart chakra, which is desirable if immune system function is disturbed.

EXERCISE

Spiral Meditation

1. With the client lying on the back, begin by placing the hands over the heart center. Following a clockwise flow, draw the spiral pattern on the full body, pausing approximately 1 minute over each energy center.

2. The sequence moves from the heart center to the solar plexus, to the high heart, down to the spleen, to the abdomen, up to the throat, then to the root, brow, knees, crown, ankles, finishing with the transpersonal point above the head.

3. Occasionally, this pattern can be modified by letting one hand follow the other hand. For example, place the right hand on the heart, and when you move the right hand to the solar plexus place the left hand on the heart, thus placing both hands on the body. The healer can also do the Spiral Meditation on himself as a self-healing process.

4. While the spiral is open, complete any intervention work using specific or full body techniques.

5. To complete the technique, close the spiral with a counter-clockwise motion starting at the transpersonal point then moving to the ankles, crown, knees, brow, root, throat, abdomen, spleen, high heart, solar plexus, and ending at the heart center. The closing of the spiral can also be done quickly by lightly touching each point.

Double Hand Chakra Balance

A technique to energize a specific chakra is to hold the hands, left over right, for a period of three minutes directly on the energy vortex. Starting with the root center, move to the sacral chakra below the navel; next, hold the solar plexus chakra at the pit of the stomach, and follow with the heart, the throat, the brow, and the crown. A music tape such as *Spectrum Suite* (Halpern, 1979) is useful as it plays 3 minutes of music in the musical key that matches each chakra. Add imagery to this procedure by using the color red for the root chakra, orange for the sacral, yellow for the solar plexus, green for the heart, blue for the throat, indigo for the brow, and violet for the crown center. This creates 21 minutes of deep relaxation and balances the energy centers. This is an ideal self-help process you can teach clients using a musical tape of their choice.

A supplemental Double Hand Balancing can be done on any area of the body over a minor chakra point anytime there is a need for reducing pain. If one is aware at the first sign that a center is closing down, this double hand boost can be used instantly to restore balance. Teach this simple and effective technique for clients to use on themselves daily and between visits to help strengthen their energy centers.

Connecting the Chakras

After assessment of the energy field and the chakra system, determine which chakra needs to be energized the most. Place one hand on the selected chakra and the other hand on the chakra above it. This connects the two chakras and will bring the vibration to a higher frequency, like plugging into a storage battery. Hold the hands in place until you feel the vibrational pattern change and the energy increase, usually in 1 to 3 minutes. Continue to hold the identified chakra and move the upper hand to the next chakra above and hold until the energy stabilizes. Continue to do this until you connect the crown chakra to the identified chakra. Then work with the chakra below, connecting it in the same manner until all of the major chakras have been connected to the identified one.

For example, if you have found that the solar plexus chakra is blocked, place your right hand on the third chakra and your left hand on the fourth chakra, holding for several minutes. Then, still holding the solar plexus chakra, move your left hand to the throat center. Hold again until it feels complete, then move the left hand to the brow, then to the crown. To work down the body, continue to hold the solar plexus chakra, but with your left hand, and move the right hand to the second chakra, then to the first chakra. Each time notice the balancing and changes that occur.

Pyramid Technique

The Pyramid technique was shown to Janet Mentgen in meditation as a way of connecting the major chakra centers with the arms and legs. It may be done by one healer, but is even more powerful with two healers. Each position is held for 1 to 3 minutes or until the client's field is smooth and flowing.

When doing this technique with two healers, each person places a hand on the root chakra, one hand on top of the other's, and each person places another hand on the hip. This forms a dynamic triangle. Proceed through the body connecting the abdomen with the knees, the solar plexus with the ankles, the throat with the shoulder, the brow with the elbows, and the crown with the wrists. Complete with all four hands on the heart.

The Pyramid technique seems to powerfully change the energy vortices and to integrate them almost as if you were adding an electrifying current. Use this when a power boost is needed for clients with weakened conditions, fatigue, or diseases such as cancer and AIDS where the immune system is depleted. This can also be used for structural problems in the musculoskeletal system.

EXERCISE

Pyramid Technique

1. Place the hand on the root chakra above the pubic bone and the other hand on the hip. Hold this position for several minutes, then move the hand from one hip to the other hip, leaving the hand in place on the root center. With this you are drawing a triangular configuration on the body.

2. Move the upper hand to the abdomen, on the second chakra, and the lower hand to the knee and hold. Move the lower hand to the other knee. Notice the triangles you are creating.

3. Move the upper hand to the solar plexus and the lower hand to one ankle and hold. Move to the other ankle and hold.

4. Move to the upper body, placing one hand above the throat center and the other hand first on one shoulder, then on the other shoulder.

5. Move the upper hand to the brow center and hold the lower hand on one elbow, then on the other elbow.

6. Move the upper hand to the crown. With the lower hand hold one wrist, then the other wrist.

7. Place both hands on the heart and hold until the process of balancing feels complete.

Lymphatic Drain

To do the Lymphatic Drain accurately, it is helpful to have a picture of the lymphatic system with you, or to remember how the system drains in the physical body. The Lymphatic Drain is a form of energetic release used to help relieve congestion and pain in the lymph system or in autoimmune diseases, such as lupus erythematosus or rheumatoid arthritis. The symptoms described by the client are generalized soreness and achiness; tenderness in the groin and neck or under the arms; and pain in the feet, ankles, and wrists.

Figure 9.2 shows the steps in numbered fashion as they are described in the Lymphatic Drain exercise. Remember to use short, brisk strokes to cleanse the energy field of congestion and follow with time for the client to rest in order to let the field realign itself.

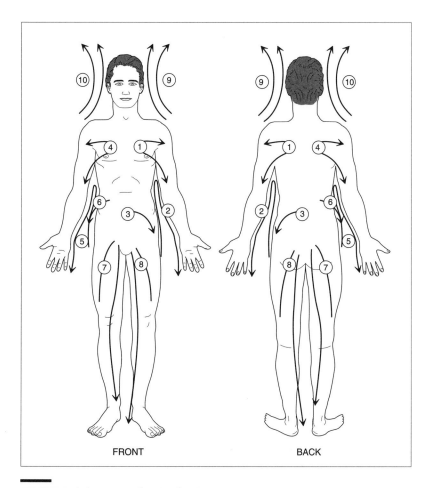

FRONT   BACK

FIGURE 9.2   Lymphatic drain.

This technique may take considerable time, from 10 to 30 minutes depending on the client's needs, but is very effective for clearing chronic and acute lymphatic congestion. It is another technique that works well with two healers working simultaneously.

EXERCISE

Lymphatic Drain

1. Begin by holding the fingers spread in a relaxed and raking position. You are going to drag your fingers against the etheric lymphatic layer, pulling across and down the body. Start raking on one side of the chest from the sternum and across the breast, continuing to do the short, rapid, raking motions until there is no longer any drag or thickness felt. The cleared field will feel light and flowing to the client.

2. Follow the same technique by placing the client's arms slightly away from the body and raking under the arms, then down the arms and off the fingers. These are short, quick pulling strokes, done rapidly, one section at a time.

3. Go to the abdomen and pull across the abdomen and off the body.

4–6. Go to the other side of the body and repeat the raking pattern in the chest, underarm areas, and abdomen.

7–8. Rake the area above the groin, down the legs, and off the foot. Repeat on the other side.

9–10. Go the head and rake up each side of the neck and the face to move congestion away from the head.

11. Turn the patient over and repeat the process on the back starting with the heart area (see numbered procedure on figure 9.2).

12. Conclude by letting the client rest, allowing time for integration and any sharing.

Technique for Sensing the Pain Ridge

When a person is experiencing acute pain, a ridge or bulge that corresponds to the pain can be found in the energetic field. This ridge may be sensed by the healer at some distance from the body, usually 12 to 18 inches away, but sometimes, as in the case of migraine headaches, it can be felt as far as 10 to 20 feet away. As you scan the field to sense the pain ridge, it usually feels warm, hot, or congested and you may sense tension or vibration in your hand.

Once you have found the ridge simply unruffle the area until it is smoothed out. Scan the energy field again, unruffling the ridge for several more minutes if needed, and then rescan. The ridge will begin to recede. Repeat this process until you can bring your hand all the way to the client's body and touch the skin without having the client report pain. This technique has been successfully used by Janet Mentgen and other Healing Touch practitioners on trigeminal neuralgia, TMJ syndrome, migraine headaches, and fractured bones. If the ridge persists, the Magnetic Pain Drain may also be used by placing the left hand on the pain ridge to siphon off the pain with the right hand.

Technique for Sealing a Wound

Whenever the body has experienced trauma, has been cut, or has given birth, the energy field, as well as the physical body, is impacted. Scan the area above the scar or injury with the palm of your hand to determine if there are any *leaks* in the energy field at the site. The leaks or breaks in the field may feel like a column of cool air, as if you are feeling a leaking inner tube. A clue that a leak is present is when a client describes a scar as remaining sore or tender for years after injury or surgery. Another symptom is a continual feeling of fatigue following a traumatic or surgical experience.

To determine whether there is such an energetic hole, check any old incisions, drainage points, or puncture sites by assessing with a hand scan or by unruffling over the scar area. To seal the leak, gather energy from the field around the area by moving your hands with the palms toward the client's skin area, back and forth over the identified spot. Then seal this extra energy supply to the skin with the palm of your hand and hold for a minute. The sealing may sound like plastic touching a hot plate with a hiss. After the area is sealed, rescan to see if any other leaks can still be detected. The area should feel as smooth and balanced as the rest of the body.

SUMMARY

Numerous interventions used by the healer during energy-based work are spontaneous and seem to be directed or guided, happening at an appropriate moment. Sometimes the intervention comes as an inner voice speaking to you, emerges as an image, or feels as if your hands are being pulled unexpectedly to a specific area of the healee's body. At other times, you may try to remove your hands and the magnetic pull is so great that it is almost impossible to lift them. So you remain awhile longer, holding the area until the hands can move freely. You may also feel intuitively drawn to sweep the area with unruffling of the energy field or placing hands on the area. The important thing is to listen to this inner guidance and to observe the outcomes.

All of the techniques described in this chapter lend themselves to precise intervention for specific client needs in almost any setting. Usually, 15 to 20 minutes is ample time to do one or several of these processes in combination. The healer needs the knowledge and skill to center, plan, implement, and evaluate the procedure. All of the techniques can be done with the client fully clothed and in a variety of clinical situations. Thus, the Healing Touch interventions offer a useful complement to other treatments the client is receiving and can be integrated unobtrusively into many helping practices, as we shall see in part 4.

References

Halpern, S. (1979). *Spectrum suite*. Belmont, CA: Halpern Sounds.

Hover-Kramer, D. (1993, March). A nurse's meditation. *Journal of Holistic Nursing, XI* (1), 115–116.

Joy, B. (1979). *Joy's way* (pp. 191–196). Los Angeles: J. P. Tarcher, Inc.

10

SPECIFIC INTERVENTIONS FOR IDENTIFIED PROBLEMS

Janet Mentgen, BSN, RN

All body systems are affected by how we think, what we eat, how we behave, and the choices we make. It is when we recognize and acknowledge our body-mind connection that we begin to awaken the healer within.

Keegan, 1994

INTRODUCTION

Energy-based interventions are a complement to the client's selected medical care and support the healing abilities of the body. One important aspect of energy work is the enhanced effect of medication and chemicals within the body. The client and healer should be alert to the possibility of side effects and sensitivity reactions. Reduction of medication to lower dosages is sometimes indicated.

Selected specific interventions are presented here that can be used for some physical problems. This list is not exhaustive, but it suggests some beginning energetic approaches. Because each client's energy field is unique, you may develop your own ways of working after assessing and careful attention to intuition. This information is based on the experiences of many nurse healers and can assist you, the caregiver, when you are deciding which way to approach a client with specific health issues.

TECHNIQUES FOR IDENTIFIED PROBLEMS

Arthritis

Use a full body technique such as Magnetic Unruffle or Full Body Connection because of the systemic nature of all arthritic problems. Follow this with Ultrasound to the specific joints involved, and teach the client how to use this technique on affected joints. The intention is to reduce pain and swelling, to retard the degenerative process, and, if possible, to restore the joint to optimum functioning.

Back Problems

A series of steps are used for back problems that begin with an assessment of the energy field on the front of the body, followed by a Full Body Connection. The client is then assisted to lie prone on a massage table, preferably with a head cradle to keep the spine and neck straight. This creates a relaxed position to support further work on the back. Another option would be for the patient to lie on the side if the prone position is too uncomfortable.

The healee with acute back pain may need to be treated daily, along with other medical or complementary interventions, until the energy field in the back remains open and flowing. Treatment can be extended to every other day, graduate to every third day, and then, be given weekly until the symptoms are gone or further intervention of another kind is implemented. You will usually see the client on a weekly basis for chronic conditions.

Assessment A hand scan or assessment with a pendulum determines the energy pattern, starting at the bottom of the spine. The pendulum should rotate clockwise up the entire back, at each vertebra. Note the direction and size of the spin. A disturbance or block is indicated when the pendulum does not move or is moving at an angle other than the clockwise spin. Sometimes, the pendulum will show no motion over the entire back, denoting severe blockage.

Scan the back with the hands and feel the other layers of the field, noting changes in sensation such as heat, tingling, suction, or pressure. Then visually scan the back of the patient by standing at the foot of the table. Note the length of the legs and symmetry or asymmetry in the shape of the shoulders and hips.

Look at the position of the body, noting where it is straight or crooked. Visually scan from the head to the feet noting any imbalance between the right and left sides.

Connecting the Lower Part of the Body   The next step is to connect the back chakras of the legs by doing a partial Full Body Connection. Starting on one leg, hold the sole of the foot with the palm of one hand and the ankle with the palm of the other hand. This creates a connection of the healer's hands with the patient. Hold this position until you feel the energy flowing, pulsating, or equalizing. Then connect the ankle to the knee and the knee to the hip. Complete the other side in a similar manner, and then hold one hand on each hip. It may take a minute or two for the energy to flow and become even. Notice any differences between the legs, including movement, muscle tension, energy flow, and temperature.

Opening the Spinal Energy Flow   Open the spinal energy flow by placing one hand at the base of the patient's neck and the other hand at the base of the spine. The energy will move in a wavelike motion, back and forth, similar to a bubble in a level, which you can sense with your hands. Keep holding this position until the energy flows smoothly and evenly. In severe imbalance, you may observe that there is no response or flow of the energy, which means that other back techniques may be more effective or that additional treatment modalities are needed before the body can respond energetically.

The Vertebral Spiral Technique   The muscles of the spine are addressed by drawing clockwise and counterclockwise circles above the spinal column beginning at the base of the neck. With the first two fingers and thumb held together, simulate the Ultrasound effect by pointing toward the spine and circling rapidly at least 10–12 times over each vertebral space. At the end of the rotations over each vertebral space, the energy will collect in the palms of your hands. You can pull your hands away from the body to release the energy buildup. Taking the hands away also allows the client's energy field to reorganize itself.

The Vertebral Spiral Technique may be done by physically touching the back or working in the energy field 1–3 inches off the back. The effect is calming and relaxing to the small muscles that lie next to the spinal column. Work all the way down the spine to the coccygeal area with your spins.

Identifying Specific Vertebrae to Release Blockage   Use the pendulum or hand scan along each vertebra to locate any further blocks or problems. Do this several times to identify the specific vertebra where energy blockage occurs. If you find the energy of the back is now flowing smoothly and the pendulum shows continuous clockwise circles, the problem was probably muscular in nature and relaxation of the back muscles was sufficient. If energy blocks are still present, then proceed with the next techniques in the specific identified areas.

The Hopi Technique   The Hopi Technique from the Native American tradition has been taught in the apprentice manner for many centuries. Rudy Noel, a Denver healer, recently shared the steps with our Healing Touch program director.

EXERCISE

The Hopi Technique

1. Place three fingers of each hand on either side of the spine, opposite each other at the identified spot where the blockage occurs (see figure 10.1). Rest your hands together as this keeps

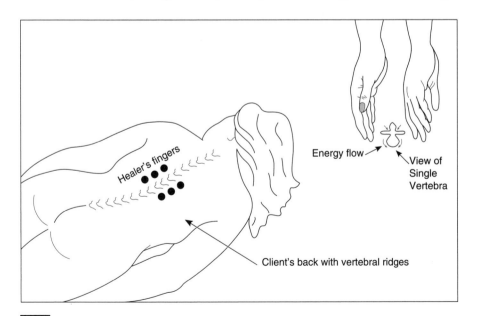

FIGURE 10.1   *The Hopi Technique, step one.*

the energy frequency running evenly. Your fingers are point-ing downward into the spine, so that the energy pours from the fingers in a laserlike fashion into the spinal column. The fingertips need to be firm on the back, and the client may feel some pressure.

2. Hold the fingers in place letting energy flow from the finger-tips into the back until pulsing occurs. Wait for a smooth, bal-anced feeling. There may be considerable vibration and your hands may shake. The key is to hold and simply stay with the vibration until it calms and becomes a gentle pulsing sensation.

3. Place both thumbs on one side of the spine closest to you and all the fingers of both hands on the opposite side of the spine as illustrated in figure 10.2. This forms an energetic ring as the etheric extensions of your fingers wrap around the spine. The energetic fingers will extend and sink inside like a claw to wrap around the spinal column. The spinal column is actually larger than what the physical hands could hold.

4. Have the client breathe deeply and experience any inner sen-sations and emotions. Images, such as events of the initial injury, may appear to the client. The client may feel pain,

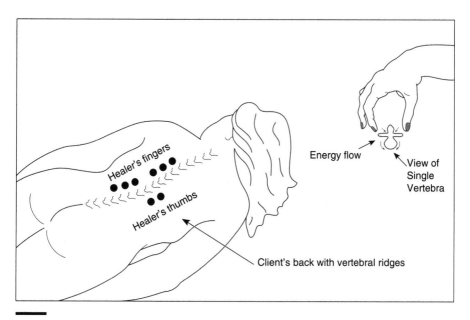

FIGURE 10.2   *The Hopi Technique, step two.*

discomfort, movement, or heat. Wait until the energy intensifies and pulsates. Breathe rhythmically with the client to establish a slower pace. When the energy connection is complete and the spine feels balanced, pull the hands rapidly straight up, breaking through the many layers of the energy field.

5. Reseal the field by placing both hands over the area of the back on which you were working. The client often feels the intensity of the energy connection and may have a sensation of temporary pressure or discomfort, which is followed by a physical or emotional release.

6. The healer can now work on other blocked areas of the back as identified by scanning. Sometimes one release will affect the whole back, and sometimes each individual area requires the Hopi Technique.

Repairing Nerve Damage   If there has been nerve damage, indicated by radiating pain following a nerve track, it is helpful to use the Laser or Ultrasound techniques by following the entire nerve. Knowledge of neuroanatomy is helpful, as well as having a mental picture of the neurological system while you are working.

Ultrasound to Repair Muscles and Joints   Ultrasound can be used on muscles and joints where pain is experienced. Often pain is referred and dependent from a spinal area; for example, the side of the hip may hurt from an energy block in the back. Always trace the entire pain track if possible.

Magnetic Pain Drain   The Magnetic Pain Drain described in chapter 9 is also effective in working with painful areas of the back.

Sweeping and Closing   On completion of the back techniques, close by placing one hand on the top of the neck and the other hand on the base of the spine. Then, holding one hand at the top, brush or sweep down and away several times to smooth the field. Have the client rise slowly and carefully. Since the energetic changes in the back take a while to be felt, wait for at least 24 hours before evaluating results of the treatment.

Focusing on the Meaning of Back Problems The back and neck are areas in which emotional issues are often stored. These need to be examined along with the physical symptoms. Common expressions about the back in our vernacular refer to emotional states. For example, we speak of feeling "strong-backed," "flexible," "stubborn," "stiff-necked," "having our back up," "carrying a cross on the back," "sticking one's neck out," "getting ahead of oneself," "looking back," "feeling backed into a corner," or "holding back." The sense of wanting to be "backed up" can represent the need for emotional, financial, or physical support. Even if you are not trained in emotional therapy, you have a responsibility to help the client explore these insights and to refer your client to psychotherapy for further treatment of major issues.

Neck Problems

Neck techniques are very similar to the procedures described for the back but require a finer and lighter touch. Remember that healing happens in the energetic body rather than by physical positioning or manipulating. With muscle relaxation the vertebrae will sometimes reposition themselves, but the goal of these techniques is the balancing of the energy field.

Begin by asking the client to relax the body and find a position in which you can comfortably reach the neck. Keeping the neck and head straight is important for energetic work. After assessing the neck to identify areas of blockage, use the Vertebral Spiral Technique over the seven small neck vertebrae. Reassess and if necessary follow with the Hopi Technique. Specific techniques, such as repairing nerve damage, Ultrasound, and Magnetic Pain Drain, may be used as indicated, followed by a complete brushing or sweeping of the energy field.

Fractured Bones

A systemic intervention, such as the Full Body Connection or Magnetic Unruffle, is helpful after any trauma to restore the balance and flow of the energy field. Use Ultrasound and unruffling over a fractured bone. Sometimes, a Laser beam into the specific area will also be helpful.

Bone Healing   The fastest bone healing witnessed by the author occurred in 48 hours, and was confirmed by X ray. The patient was treated immediately after a fracture of the humerus, midway down the arm, with 6 minutes of unruffling and Ultrasound while she was standing under a shower. She experienced very little pain and was only inconvenienced by the wearing of a splint for a week to be assured the bone was healed.

Another example was a home care client with a fractured tibia from osteoporosis that healed in 3 months. The ankle was not casted due to severe swelling and limited mobility of the patient. Codeine was used for pain control. Ultrasound to the fracture site and Full Body Connection were used 2 to 3 times a week by several home health caregivers.

A Healing Touch practitioner witnessed an unusual healing with her son who sustained a compression fracture of the back. The tips of the vertebrae at T-10, T-11, and T-12 were knocked off and could be seen floating free from the spine on X ray. He was treated with a back brace, which he wore faithfully for 2 weeks, and pain medication, of which he took only one dose. In addition, unruffling was done on his back 3 to 4 times daily for the first 2 weeks. Then he was pain-free except for occasional back strain. After he joined the navy, he was questioned about his fractured back, as evidenced from medical records. He showed no scarring or evidence of fracture on repeated X ray. Amazingly, not only were the tips of the bones back in alignment, but no scar line was visible on later X rays.

Multiple Sclerosis (MS)

People with MS or other demyelinating symptoms are unable to maintain an open energy system. The energy centers will open easily with a Full Body Connection, but they will not stay open. From our experience, it takes nearly 6 months of weekly balancing by the therapist and daily work by a family member to help the energy field to maintain a full and open flow. Symptoms seem to disappear in reverse order, with the most recent symptom disappearing first. There is usually steady but subtle improvement. Keeping written records of the release of symptoms is important in order to measure progress over such a long period of time.

Balancing the field seems to enhance any other practices the client is already doing. Energy interventions may slow down the degenerative process of the disease. The difficult part, as mentioned, is the continued repetition that is required to maintain an open field. It is helpful to teach a family member or friend to use the Full Body Connection and Magnetic Unruffle on a daily basis. Additional therapeutic interventions of imagery, focusing, and psychotherapy are also helpful.

Premenstrual Syndrome (PMS)

In persons who suffer from PMS the entire chakra system seems to go into spasm at a specific time in the menstrual cycle. Once there is a spasm, a biochemical process follows, which produces the systemic premenstrual symptoms. After the initial closing of the energy field, most treatments seem only to chase symptoms. To work with the energetic spasm, daily scanning and recording of the condition of each chakra is needed to identify specifically when a chakra shuts down so that it can be energized immediately. It may take several months of observation to determine the client's pattern.

To assist the client, balance the body fully every week with the Full Body Connection or the Double Hand Chakra Balance. The client learns to sense how an open and balanced chakra system feels and develops ways of sensing when the chakras close. After 3 to 4 months of self-observation, the client can usually identify specifically when the chakras close, which one closes first, and the specific time when this occurs. For example, the client can precisely state, "At 10:30 A.M. on day 19 of the cycle, the throat chakra closes. On day 20, three more are closed, and on day 22, I experience the systemic symptoms of bloating, irritability, and achiness." If the beginning of the energetic spasm is caught immediately, the complex symptoms of PMS may be prevented and the client can become asymptomatic.

Headaches

To work on a headache, the most common symptom of pain in our society, first identify the type of headache with which you are working. A careful history will be helpful to determine the pattern, frequency, intensity, duration, medications, and treatments used for relief.

Tension Headaches   Tension headaches are muscular in nature, and usually originate in the upper or lower back and involve the back of the neck and head. The relaxation techniques of Full Body Connection, Mind Clearing, and Therapeutic Touch are helpful to eliminate the pain.

Sinus Headaches   Sinus headaches, due to allergies, irritations, and infection, create frontal pain and may require medication as well as energy work. Direct release by balancing the crown, brow, and throat chakras, followed by Ultrasound and unruffling, seem to be most helpful. This can be repeated frequently until symptoms abate. Decongestive medication may interfere with the symptomatic relief and immediate results may be less evident,but it is wise to offer Healing Touch treatments as an adjunct to medications and to enhance the effectiveness of medications.

Migraine Headaches   Migraine headaches require a specific treatment protocol. The client should be seen weekly for a Full Body Connection and to obtain a complete history of the headache pattern. If you see the client during an acute headache, unruffle the pain ridge, which can only be done in the acute phase. This ridge often has a spike that is in the direction of the headache and can be sensed many feet away from the body. Note how the pattern of the headache begins to change and eventually stops with continued energy-balancing work. Unfortunately, most pain medication used for migraine headache relief closes the chakras and related layers of the energetic field by blocking the neuroreceptor sites.

Head Trauma   Head trauma responds best to the Full Body Connection, the Etheric Unruffle, and the Magnetic Unruffle. Repair the trauma site and the energy field around the head to restore the shape of the etheric field. Closed head injury symptoms respond with a number of energy balancing techniques over a period of 3 to 4 months.

Hypertension

The person with hypertension usually has a blocked root chakra, and the Full Body Connection is the most helpful treatment as the entire body is affected by the increased blood pressure. If the person remains on antihypertensive medication, it takes about 6 weeks before a measurable decrease in the blood pressure is noted. If the person is not medicated, there is often an immediate, measurable response of blood pressure drop during the energetic treatment. To work successfully with blood pressure reduction over the long term, encourage the lifestyle changes needed in addition to weekly energy balancing and self-care techniques. Lifetime monitoring of blood pressure is recommended. Many healers also use biofeedback tapes and relaxation training as additional therapies.

PRE- AND POSTOPERATIVE TECHNIQUES

Prior to surgery, see the patient for an energetic balancing and relaxation training. The more prepared the person is for the surgical intervention, the easier the surgical experience usually is. It makes a significant difference if the client enters the surgical procedure in a relaxed and balanced state, rather than in a tired, stressed, or fearful condition. Relaxation can happen very rapidly with the Full Body Connection or Magnetic Unruffle.

Instruct the client to tell the anesthesiologist that he is working with energetic approaches and may require less anesthesia. This is to prevent toxicity from overuse of medication. Also, encourage the patient to request having meditation tapes in the operating and recovery rooms and to limit all conversation to positive suggestions for healing. Remember that the unconscious mind hears and takes in literally everything that is said in the surgical arena.

The hospital staff may not understand or be supportive of these approaches, mostly due to lack of knowledge. It is the patient's right to have what he wants in the hospital setting, which includes an environment that is conducive to healing.

Postoperatively, the patient needs to be balanced fully to restore the energetic flow and to release any of the anesthesia trapped in the cellular tissues. Use the Magnetic Unruffle to release the chemicals, smooth the energy over the surgical site, and then gather energy for sealing the wound. Seal any puncture holes in the skin and don't forget the holes in the energy field left by drainage tubes. Energize the IV bottle and solution by holding your hands around the bottle and tubing, and energize all medication and dressings with your hands and intention.

Teach the patient how to unruffle the site before blood is drawn and to unruffle any area where IM or IV medication is injected. Nausea is helped by unruffling and balancing the solar plexus chakra.

Pain Control

For pain control, instruct the client in self-care techniques, such as unruffling or moving the energetic Ultrasound around painful areas. Discuss how the patient can ask for pain medication if needed and how to refuse medication if it is not needed. Hospital personnel sometimes medicate using protocols for the general public rather than addressing the individual needs of the patient. Family members can help by using the Chakra Spread for relaxation, transferring energy to painful areas, and massaging the feet.

MEDICAL PROCEDURES

Here are some simple hints to help reduce pain and anxiety before, during, and after invasive medical procedures. Before inserting a nasogastric tube, unruffle the throat area and make sure you as the caregiver are centered. Before beginning an intravenous infusion, unruffle over the site to be punctured. The vein will not roll, will stand up nicely for you, and the procedure will not cause pain. To remove a needle, unruffle the area as you hold the site with cotton and pressure. Smooth or unruffle any treatment site to relieve pain and help medication to absorb more readily. Transfer energy from the Universal Energy Field to assist the patient at any time during a procedure by simply placing the hands on or above the procedure site.

SUMMARY

As can be seen, there are numerous direct applications of Healing Touch for medical problems. There is not sufficient space to go into all of them in detail, but this presentation gives you some ideas about ways to begin. As you find an approach that is helpful to the client, other techniques and intuitive ways of working with the client's energy field will often come to you.

The rapid relaxation that occurs with the energy-based techniques allows you as the caregiver to be genuinely present to assist the patient. The emotional impact of these interventions is increased trust and rapport between the healer and the client. And patients are often delighted to find that they can participate in preventing their own discomfort. This sense of self-control and mastery of the environment is often a most significant outcome because patients and staff alike are trying to cope with the impersonal, mechanized settings that characterize most hospitals and clinics.

Reference

Keegan, L. (1994). *The nurse as healer* (p. 77). Albany, NY: Delmar Publishers, Inc.

11 | THE CLINICAL PRACTICE OF HEALING TOUCH

Janet Mentgen, BSN, RN

> *Healing Touch is the art of caring that comes from the heart of the healer and reaches to the person who is receiving help.*
>
> Janet Mentgen

INTRODUCTION

Healing happens within the client as the body returns to a state of energetic balance. From an energy-based perspective, physical or mental disease is understood as imbalance or disharmony in the client's entire energy field. It is the work of caregivers and health care professionals to assist in the restoration of balance. This is accomplished by creating a healing environment and by facilitating connection with the client's own healing potential. The outcome of an intervention from a helper may be full restoration of balance in the field, partial regaining of balance (which means accepting some areas of imbalance), or physical death with the possibility of expansion in the other layers of the energy field.

A healer must trust that what occurs in this subtle, noninvasive work is for the highest good of the individual. The energy that the healer helps to make available will be used in the way that is most needed by the client. This means that we do not really know what the best outcome would be from our limited perspectives and that we must learn to operate from the larger picture that includes the client's inner world. We always heal from the place of neutral detachment, letting go of any personal attachment to outcomes. This does not mean withdrawal or indifference but rather a state of being centered and fully present and releasing personal investment in the client's choice or path. As healers we learn to help as we can and to leave without comment so that the healing process can unfold without interference. This allows the wisdom of the client's inner healing power to emerge.

In this chapter we will explore the qualities and development of the healer that allow this kind of practice to happen. We will further discuss how the healing environment can be established and will delineate the steps of a Healing Touch treatment sequence. Finally, we will briefly describe the practice of Healing Touch that is evolving with national recognition of healing work.

THE HEALER

Attributes of a Healer

The healer's intent is to help someone in need and to see the person in wholeness. This means that there is a sense of commitment and focus on what is best for the healee. The response of the healer becomes automatic in situations of need and may range from performing an actual Healing Touch procedure to simply imaging the client in health while sending the pure intent of caring. There may be hundreds of opportunities to assist others when we are open and flexible.

The healer's ability to center is essential. Centering is the focused intent that is required to hold a point of reference, which is the connection with the soul and the Universal Energy Field through the head, heart, and hands. In addition, the healer's physical body needs to be relaxed, the emotions calm, the mind clear of tension, and the spirit quiet and still. Thus, maintaining a personal state of wellness and vitality and minimizing stresses whenever possible becomes the ongoing preparation of the healer.

Other qualities of the healer include spontaneous compassion for the client, a sense of self-confidence, trust in the resources of the universe, and a firm knowledge and skill base. The abilities to use imagery, to guide others and to creatively bring ideas together are other helpful attributes. As we develop these essentials and share with our clients, there is a sense of joy and personal satisfaction.

Development of a Healer

How does one learn to be a healer? There is often an identifiable learning sequence. It may begin with a life event, a loss or a serious illness, that drives us into new ways of thinking. Our personal experience becomes a great teacher; the perceived crisis becomes an opportunity for stretching and exploring new possibilities. As we open with increasing curiosity to whatever presents itself, we notice what works and what does not to facilitate the restoration of health and harmony. Then we move beyond our personal boundaries to apply what we have learned in helping others.

The Choice The choice to work in one of the healing arts may be made consciously after resolving a personal crisis, or it may be made subconsciously out of the desire to heal oneself. Many people in the healing professions today experience frustration in their work because they are unable to fully express their creative wish to help others. Another part of the frustration among health caregivers comes from unresolved personal issues that may have attracted us to becoming helpers early in life.

To become a genuine healer means making a serious commitment to self-knowledge and compassion for others. In other words, the choice to work in a health-related field is merely a beginning. Facing one's doubts, fears, past traumas, and personal shadow is part of the development needed. Self-awareness and confidence also protect the client from misguided projections and assist the healer to set clear boundaries and stay unobtrusive. Learning to be a healer, then, requires development of oneself with experience, openness, and discipline. We will deal more fully with the vital issues of self-care and personal growth of the healer in part 5.

Study Healing work demands diligent study of the art and science of healing. Knowledge of anatomy, physiology, the emotional and mental dimensions, social and medical science, intuition, counseling, and a personal sense of spiritual connection

— are all essential. There is literally no end to the information we can gather, or the classes we can attend, to become proficient in assisting others. Fortunately, we do not have to wait to be an accomplished expert. We grow with the process of questioning and exploring, initially learning from other healers who have the expertise, and then letting our own experience become the teacher and guide.

Practice   In addition to studying, begin to practice with family members, friends, animals, and plants before tackling strangers and patients. No matter how awkward the beginning, practice, practice, and more practice is essential to sense energy in your hands. Practice feeling the energy fields around others, sick or well, in order to identify how human energy responds. Practice sensing the energy field whenever anyone calls your attention to pain, discomfort, injury, or emotional distress, and you will quickly learn to identify the differences from a pain-free field.

Most important is the intuitive knowing to pause, listen, and respond before taking any action. Healers spend much time learning to be fully in the here and now, in the moment, when the world stops and opens to the present. Awareness of clients' needs comes from being fully present and attuned to their energy. Then, your body quickens, like an antenna going up and rotating in all directions to pick up the cues. Only after this careful attuning do you move into action. You can proceed without doubt; you know intuitively just what to do. Sometimes you are drawn to a location in a client's energy field without cognitive perception. It is as if you are guided to do the healing work once you have paid attention to all the preparatory steps.

CREATING A HEALING ENVIRONMENT

It is not easy for a person who is in pain or who is experiencing fear to trust that physical or emotional sensations can be released. The distress of serious illness or panic from loss of control of the physical body can cause frustration, disappointment, and discouragement and create severe tension. The work of the healer is to help create an environment that assists the client to experience relaxation in the body, to release emotional attachments and the need for control in every situation, and to develop an attitude of hope and surrender.

Ideally, the healing environment is one of simple beauty that encourages feelings of safety and protection. This may not always be possible in health care settings, so it is even more important to build rapport through your caring, gentleness, honesty, and support. Enter the client's energy field with softness, as any rough or quick movement is jarring and may create more pain and discomfort. For the client, receiving your healing touch is like being held, rocked, and caressed. This kind of sensation allows the client to surrender so that energy repatterning to wholeness can happen. Healing begins when the client's body rebuilds itself because no tension or blockage stands in the way. This can happen best when the healer is centered and the healee is relaxed.

Observers are often present, such as students, family, or other professionals. As the healer and healee center and attune, the awareness of others seems to disappear. The more experienced you are, the less self-conscious you will feel about doing Healing Touch with others present. Another option is to invite the observers to add their centering, interest, intent, and caring to the effectiveness of the work.

As already implied, the work must be done in an atmosphere of complete trust. The healer learns to trust his inner, subtle perceptions; the client trusts the knowledge and skills of the healer; they both trust that the appropriate outcomes will emerge. Confidentiality is, of course, essential.

HEALING TOUCH SESSIONS

Although many Healing Touch interventions can be given in a few moments in busy hospital settings, the ideal is a 1-hour healing session that can be scheduled privately at the client's convenience. By following a plan such as the one outlined, you will be able to work in an organized way. Documentation of the interventions used also assists treatment planning, especially if the client comes several times. Needless to say, all client records are kept secure and private in a locked filing system.

Steps in Healing Touch Sessions

Initial Interview   The initial interview provides the working base for energetic interventions and functions as an intake assessment. A data sheet is needed to record enough information about the client's initial status to make effective comparisons later. You will find a sample intake sheet in Appendix A.

The first contact with the client is an important occasion. Introduce yourself and explain enough about your work so that a feeling of confidence can begin to develop. Determine the reasons the client has come, asking for data about the problem. All data you collect about the client assists you in determining his energetic patterns. To this end, relevant medical history, hospitalizations, diseases, injuries, and diagnoses, as well as medication history, are helpful. Ask about current medications, including recreational drugs, alcohol, caffeine, nicotine, vitamins, and herbs, as their ingestion may significantly impact the energy field.

It is helpful to determine which layer of the field is most important to the client's self-perception so that your treatment plan can directly address the needs of the client. The client's most perceived concerns may be in the physical, emotional, mental, or spiritual dimension or in combinations of several dimensions. The client may speak of feeling "scattered," "dense," "spacey," "together," or use metaphorical expressions, like "I've been dragging around," "I feel pushed," or "I'm getting ahead of myself." These phrases of speech give clues to current stresses in the personal or professional life that you can further explore.

Look at major issues in lifestyle, relationships, perceptions, and goals. Over time, stress can build to cause repeated deficits in the energy field and the onset of physical symptoms. It is also useful to find out which areas of the person's life are going smoothly. Information about relaxation and play will tell you how the client nurtures himself and paces his lifestyle and awareness to self-caring activities. In the current time of public interest in self-improvement, many clients come with experience in support groups, self-hypnosis, meditation, 12-step programs, imagery, daily exercise, and nutritional planning. All of the things the client is already doing can become valuable resources as you plan your interventions.

It is important to make note of other health care professionals — physicians, psychologists, chiropractors, body-oriented therapists, counselors — that are working with the client. For ethical and legal purposes, you should assure that the client is receiving adequate medical care. If the client is, in your opinion, not adequately served, then referrals and strong recommendations should be made as Healing Touch is always a complementary approach. Another reason for determining the client's other professionals is for networking and developing understanding of your work in the community.

Listen to what the client's body is telling you. The body is a perfect feedback system if we allow ourselves to pay attention. From the holistic perspective, discomfort and malfunction are signals that something further is needed for wholeness. Although traditional medical approaches may be to cut out or remove the broken part, the energetic view is to learn from the symptoms. Pain, for example, is a useful signal, much like a fire alarm. If we simply eliminate the pain with medication, we get a temporary solution, like taking the batteries out of the fire alarm. In the long run this removal of symptoms does not help us to deal with the underlying problem. However, if we ask when, how often, and under what circumstances the pain occurs, we can learn how to prevent its onset or minimize the distress. The body is the receiver of all the energetic forces coming from the environment; it does not create the problem. We might ask, then, not so much what the specific problems are but rather which client, with certain energetic and stress patterns, has this particular problem.

Assessment   Assessment of the energy field with the hands is like an interview, only done with the hands. Our bodies are symmetrical and should feel the same on both sides. In wellness, the energy flows evenly from head to toe without blocks, breaks, unevenness, or temperature variations. Any disruption of the flow reflects disharmony in that area and suggests the need for further exploration.

Approach the client from a centered state, releasing any preconceived ideas about what you might find. Determine the shape of the energy field by slowly scanning its outer edges. Start 3 to 4 feet away from the body and move toward it using the palms as sensors. Continue until you can determine the actual outline of the energy field.

The ways that energy is sensed in the field include temperature differentials, ridges over painful areas, blockage of energy flow, disorganized patterns, magnetic pulls, or protective armoring. Pain may feel like needles, prickly, buzzing, or shooting darts. Blocks may feel still, sluggish, heavy, hollow, sticky, or compacted. Disorganized energy feels rough, bumpy, static, or ruffled with whorls of erratic flows. Magnetic pulls feel like depletion, emptiness, sucking, grasping, pushing, or pulling. Protective armoring has very definite boundaries and serves to encapsulate or protect a vulnerable area.

The healer continues the assessment by feeling the vital layer of the field, 1 to 6 inches off the skin, and by moving toward the body. The chakras in the palms of the hands are the receptors that pick up differences in temperature and pressure and other information. These receptors sense warmth and coolness that is quite different from the physical temperature of the hand, which you can test by placing your hand on the client's skin.

As you sense the energy field, you are usually aware of temperature differences first, and then you begin to notice pulsation, vibrations, or turbulence. Remember to be very alert, as changes are subtle and may happen quickly even as you are assessing. You want to be able to identify areas in relation to the physical body where the field is different, perhaps not as vibrant or as smooth as in other areas.

Note also the energy of each chakra or center as described in chapter 5. Each chakra has its own unique vibrational pattern and will feel different from the field as a whole. With experience you will be able to detect the chakras as you move your hands over the vortices since the sensation feels like something is brushing your hand. Comparison can be made between the centers so that you can determine which ones are open and which ones are blocked, unable to receive the flow from the Universal Energy Field.

Documentation   Documentation of the assessment begins with the initial client contact and continues throughout the entire visit. Mentally make note of all sensations, even the ones that may seem very subtle. You may need to devise your own vocabulary for these subtle perceptions, such as "full," "empty," "dense," because of the subjective nature of the observations. A picture of the energy pattern is usually easy to do by drawing the perceived pattern on a simple outline of the body. Areas of energetic differences can be drawn in as can injuries, swelling, scars, or the track of a pain ridge. Colors can be added to denote areas where you sensed color, especially in relation to the chakras. Brightness or dullness are other ways that we visually distinguish the differences between blocked and open centers.

Intervention   The healer can choose many healing interventions in the sequence, such as the ones described in earlier chapters. The art of healing comes in being able to make intelligent choices for the greatest effectiveness. The more the healer can learn about the various energetic modalities, the wiser the choice she can make. During the intervention time, which may last 20 to 30 minutes, all of the healer's skill and prior experience is utilized. Thus, knowledge of counseling or of issues the client might encounter when in an altered state of consciousness add further depth to the healing work.

Completion and Grounding   After completion of the interventions, carefully ground the client. One way to do this is to hold the feet until you sense a flow and connection with the client and sense that the client's energy is back in the feet. Another way is to brush down the body from head to toe and down the arms toward the ground. Do this briskly several times. Often, clients will spontaneously start moving their hands and feet as they reconnect fully with the body. You may also choose to give a suggestion, "Feel your fingers, and your toes; now gently move them until you return to full awareness in this room."

After suggesting a return to awareness in the present, spend some time with the client to obtain feedback. Focus on what the client experienced, helping him to stay with the immediacy of the moment. Note what you sensed as the client describes his process. Talking helps the client to feel grounded as well. Carefully determine that the client is fully alert before allowing him to leave. It is also useful to reassess the energy field at this time and to document the changes.

Follow-up Visits   One healing sequence is sometimes adequate for a client to achieve her goals, but frequently more than one session is indicated. For long-term or chronic problems, considerable repatterning of the energy field is needed on a weekly basis. If the person has acute symptoms, more frequent visits may be necessary to help hold the energy field open. Teaching the client's family members or friends specific interventions that you found most helpful is a good way to enhance the time between visits. If medical treatment is also being given, make sure you get laboratory findings and test reports to monitor progress. Also, be aware of the need to adjust medications if side effects develop. Overall, let the client's responses to your energetic interventions determine the rate of progress, and set a schedule that seems logical to you.

Completion of the Work   Discharge planning begins with the initial visit as the goals of the healing work are set. The end objective is to find the optimum choices for the client and to have the resource people available for this through referrals. Although complete well-being is our hope, this may not be possible within our human time frame. Sometimes there is an obvious need for surgical intervention, and the healer can assist by preparing the client and offering support throughout the surgical process. At other times, the need for psychotherapy is evident, and the healer would refer unless she is also a qualified therapist.

If the client is no longer in need of energetic intervention but wishes to maintain the contact for prevention and health enhancement, a more relaxed schedule can evolve. In such a case, the client determines the pacing of visits unless there is a change in the client's condition that requires more frequent visits.

THE HEALING TOUCH PRACTITIONER

Most practitioners of energy-based therapies enter the field with a basic education in a health care profession like nursing, counseling, or massage. Depending on their state's licensing laws related to touching clients for a fee, they can add the specific training in Healing Touch to their credentials and proceed to practice. Non-health professionals can work privately within the family setting, assisting others as a first aid intervention, as part of a healing ministry, and for self-care, always within the scope of adequate medical care. If nonprofessionals wish to do Healing Touch in a more public way, they need to obtain the appropriate education and licensure required in their state.

The Healing Touch program, which is offered through the American Holistic Nurses' Association, has recently added certification as a way of acknowledging persons who have gone through the carefully sequenced educational and mentorship process. The criteria for certification of these practitioners are listed in appendix B. It usually takes 2 to 3 years even for very mature and committed individuals to complete the program and apply for certification.

The true significance of national recognition of energy-based healing rests in the future. This is the first time that a mainstream, medically related organization has acknowledged healers and their skills. Much will depend on the insight and wisdom that the new Healing Touch practitioners demonstrate and their ability to communicate their talents effectively to others. Ultimately, the consumer who experiences the work will determine its value and seek out the newly recognized, certified healers.

SUMMARY

We see now how the careful preparation of the healer becomes the foundation of a dynamic, integrated practice. As we have stated, balancing of the energy field is a necessary complement to other modalities, like psychotherapy, massage, body-oriented approaches, and traditional medical practice. We might think of energy work as the missing piece in the current health care picture. We will explore the vital linkages with other disciplines in the next section.

HEALING TOUCH PRACTICE AS A COMPLEMENT TO OTHER HELPING MODALITIES

As we have suggested throughout the book, Healing Touch is a modality that best serves as a complement or an adjunct to other modalities. In the next three chapters we will explore the ways in which this energetic work enhances the traditional practices of medicine, body-oriented therapies, and psychotherapy.

BRIDGES WITH
MEDICAL AND
CLINICAL SETTINGS

*Local theories of the mind are not only incomplete,
they are destructive. They create the illusion of death
and aloneness, altogether local concepts. They foster
existential oppression and hopelessness by giving us
an utterly false idea of our basic nature. . . . This
local scenario is ghastly, and it is regrettable that it
continues to dominate the picture put forth by most
of our best psychologists and bioscientists.*

Dossey, L., 1989

INTRODUCTION

As the chapter quote suggests, the medical profession and its
related helping professionals have defined their expertise too nar-
rowly. By focusing exclusively on the physical realm, opportunities
for the kind of closure I experienced with little Paul's family (chapter 1) are missed. At a time when the family genuinely needed a
steady, caring professional, they felt abandoned because the physicians had limited their ministrations to ways of helping Paul stay
alive. When this became impossible, they apparently withdrew and
left the family to fend for themselves.

Larry Dossey, MD is an internist with many years of experience who writes about ways this misplaced concreteness severely

limits and constricts the work of bioscientists (Dossey, 1982). Over and over in medical practice one meets the exceptional patient who improves despite the worst prognosis as well as the person who expires when she has given up hope. In constricting our understanding to a local view, i.e., the mind is contained in the physical brain, we also see death as the ultimate end and, therefore, the enemy. When we begin to see consciousness as infinite, in a nonlocal way, then moral, ethical, and spiritual considerations become more important. We may, for example, begin to talk about the quality of life that a certain technology can give rather than unquestioningly utilizing life-prolonging measures. Or we may consider the ways in which the patient can heal emotionally to have a positive and conscious death.

FROM PARTS TO THE WHOLE

Other physicians and thinkers are writing about these more expanded views of the mind as well. A family practitioner who works with Native American populations in the Southwest has found that physicians are empowered beings, like the priests of the past, who can help persuade the individual to heal. "If belief helps a patient to find comfort, and if we believe we can help patients, then we must invoke the power of all healing sacraments to do so — to help the patient grow and heal, or even to accept losses and death" (Hammerschlag, 1989, p. 87). In learning to become a healer, he found that patients do not need a scientist who simply carries out instructions but rather a caring person who helps them to find connections between themselves and their inner being, and between themselves and something greater than science.

Scientific Changes and Progress

In a more scientific vein, Richard Gerber, MD, addresses the basis for a new paradigm of medical practice in *Vibrational Medicine* (1988). The shift in science from the atomic, fragmented Newtonian worldview to the unbroken wholeness of Einstein and the quantum mechanical worldview is gradually impacting every part of our lives. This includes how we see the body, its relation to mind, and the universe in which we live. Gerber's book elaborates in detail how healing, via systems that affect the subtle energies, is an extension of existing medical science just as the Einsteinian viewpoint is an extension of the Newtonian physics. If all matter is really energy, as Einstein insists, then we must see the human body as a dynamic, interactive energy system and develop ways to work with this energy for healing.

Whether individual bioscientists and medical practitioners believe this new model of the world or not is relatively unimportant. The facts are that science is progressing rapidly beyond our wildest fantasies. The effectiveness of existing medical technology is constantly enhanced by new, adjunctive discoveries. The MRI (magnetic resonance imaging), for example, is energetic in principle. The atoms under study, usually hydrogen, are stimulated by the transfer of energy at a specific frequency. The energy is only absorbed by the atom if it is of a particular resonant frequency such as that of healthy cells. Thus, an energetic picture of the area to be studied unfolds giving the analyst images of healthy and defective structure in the tissues (Gerber, 1988, pp. 104–106).

Other research in the field of neurotransmitters and neuropeptides points to the complex interactions of the body and mind. It is no longer enough to look at the isolated parts of neuroanatomy because the whole is apparently much more than the sum of its parts. Although the hard sciences have largely ignored consciousness and intuition, the physical body is now understood to be exquisitely connected to thought and hunches. The body matches our thought patterns instantly through the biochemical changes within the neuropeptides and their receptors (Pert, 1986) and we can accurately speak of *bodymind* as one integrated concept.

Another sign of change within medical thinking is the tremendous public response that Deepak Chopra, MD, has received in speaking about Ayurvedic medicine based on age-old Indian traditions. In a time of highly developed medical technologies, Chopra found his spirit hungry despite high achievements as an endocrinologist and as chief of staff at a New England hospital. He turned to learning from the inner wisdom of the body, "the organizing power that flows from its deep source in the self and coordinates every aspect of the physical system" (1991, p. 202). Meditation is the vehicle for accessing this inner wisdom. Meditation or centering focuses the mind, but it also permits activation of the parasympathetic nervous system's responses and the biochemical changes that produce endorphins and increase functioning of the immune system (Chopra, 1990).

Complementary Practices

The times seem ripe for numerous complementary approaches to augment the tremendous strides that have been made in the biochemical sciences. These complementary practices can enhance medical practice by incorporating the energetic model of quantum physics, the bodymind understanding of psychoneuroimmunology, and the holistic view of interacting systems that are much more than their individual parts.

HEALING TOUCH AS A COMPLEMENTARY APPROACH

Healing Touch can rightly be seen as one of these complementary approaches. As the following examples show, there are many applications in hospital and clinical settings that allow the patient to receive the best possible care, not only physically but emotionally, and at more subtle energetic levels. Thus, Healing Touch can extend the medical practitioner's treatment to include aspects that could not be addressed by traditional means. Finding ways that the client can extend his self-care and become an active participant in improving health (Coleman & Gurin, 1993) is an essential component of modern medical care. Healing Touch offers excellent resources for such self-care and thus becomes a viable adjunct to clinical care.

Pre- and Postprocedural Care

Many medical procedures, including surgery, chemotherapy, and complex diagnostic testing, produce anxiety in the client, even prior to their onset. A simple Healing Touch technique like the Magnetic Unruffle done 5 minutes before the procedure, can help the client to feel less distraught and remind him of his internal resources for coping with stress. An energy field technique combined with relaxation imagery can be even more powerful so that preoperative medication can be kept to a minimum.

In the time after a medical procedure, smoothing of the energy field, especially at the intervention site is necessary. Assessment of the field by hand scan or penduling often shows that the area is depleted, flat, or cold in spite of the fact that a wound is physically sealed. This suggests that something further is needed to rebalance the energy flows, otherwise the client may report feeling "drained" or "fragmented" even months later.

Several Healing Touch students on the West Coast are dermatological surgeons who excise facial tumors on a daily basis. They have found unruffling the energy field a helpful way to start preoperative preparation. They find that the patient needs less local anesthesia and is more relaxed during the operation. At the end, these caring surgeons put their energy into the wound dressing and smooth the entire field before the patient leaves. Stitches can often be removed earlier than the usual 7 days because of the accelerated wound healing when Healing Touch is used.

Because of the advances of medical science, many persons are alive with severe illnesses that require repeated treatments. Kidney dialysis, for example, is repeated three times a week and can prolong life for many years until a suitable transplant is found. In spite of the wonders of this technology, many dialysis patients undergo severe personal and emotional stress related to the procedures that makes their daily life almost unbearable. The human toll in anxiety is something that medical science has few means to address. However, preprocedural fears can be diminished with Healing Touch and some of the self-care techniques suggested in chapter 15. The disarray of the person's energy field after dialysis responds well to energetic rebalancing by a family member.

Joan's Story

I recently had the opportunity to work with a young dialysis patient named Joan, whose presenting problem was a severe needle phobia that made the frequent trips to the dialysis center an unimaginable ordeal. No amount of medication or tranquilizing agent made an impact. Bit by bit, I taught Joan how to use the Ultrasound technique over the needle insertion sites and an affirmation, a repeated positive statement, to comfort her inner fears. To this we added creative imaging of peaceful scenes and pictures of the goals for which she was staying alive. Her practice was so successful that the shunt lasted for more than 5 years, a time sufficient to prepare for the impending transplant. Even though the implant operation was to take place many miles from home, Joan felt quite relaxed because, through our networks, the Healing Touch nurses from that community came to assist her before and after surgery.

Assisting with Incurable Illness

Many medical practices deal with severe, physically incurable illnesses such as cancer and AIDS. Again, it makes sense to look for other ways to assist the patient when medical science has reached its limits. "There is nothing further we can do for you" is a verdict that not only creates a feeling of hopelessness in the sufferer, but also denies the existence of many other resources.

Several new publications speak of the personality profiles of exceptional cancer patients with stage IV, widely metastatic disease. "The patients who significantly outlived their expectancy were more creative, more receptive to new ideas, flexible and argumentative. They had strong egos and expressed feelings of personal adequacy and vitality. . . . They sought out innovative medical treatment, refusing to accept the death sentence handed out with their diagnosis. In this sense, they were seen as using a form of denial — not denying the seriousness of their disease by any means, but denying that they would be victims" (Achterberg, 1985, p. 180).

Healing Touch, especially the vitalizing techniques that work from the lower body to the higher levels, gives many options for persons like this. There is plenty of time while one is dying to learn more and to complete life tasks such as relating to the family and winding up business affairs. If the client chooses to be alert and conscious, there are many insights along the way of the final earthly journey.

The Chakra Spread is, of course, the energetic treatment of choice when someone is in the final stages of dying. Often, family members feel the need to help but have no specific way to assist their loved one. The Chakra Spread technique is easy to learn and appears to be satisfying both to the patient, who is often agitated or struggling for breath, and to the family member who is helping to expand the energy field for an easy transition.

Jim's Story

Jim was a singer and dancer whose love of life bubbled over into every aspect of his terminal AIDS diagnosis. He was unwilling to accept the medical facts by quietly preparing for his death. Instead, he wanted to learn ways of making the best possible use of the little time he had.

Despite deep bouts of depression, he began to create pictures and songs out of his pain. He used the Chakra Connection on himself daily and whenever he felt tired or "out of kilter." His wife noticed how, despite his neuropathy, his mind stayed alert with the Mind Clearing Technique through the pain and physical chaos. Most importantly, Jim no longer felt powerless; he felt he had ways of dealing with the difficult times.

Jim long outlived his life expectancy, learning about his humanness and about his connections with the Higher Power. "Every day had a gift," he said before his passing. "The songs and melodies just kept coming. I hope my songs will help someone else to see their light."

Helping with Birthing and Neonates

Just as the energy-related work assists those exiting from the physical body, so it is relevant in helping people to come into earthly life. Krieger's studies with families before the birth of their child show the tremendous bonding that can happen as the couple prepares by sensing the child's and, later, the family's energy field (Krieger, 1993, pp. 138–143).

One of our practitioners is a nurse midwife we'll call Ruth. She has her own private practice and also regularly assists with births at a local hospital. From the beginning of labor until several hours after the birth, she fosters relaxation in the mothers by doing the Magnetic Unruffle and the Chakra Spread. Smoothing the baby's energy field after birth with a few short sweeps calms the little one and often brings a wide-eyed smile.

Ruth has also found Healing Touch techniques very helpful with neonates, especially those that are having some physical difficulties. Since medication is usually contraindicated, she uses unruffling over the area or Ultrasound for reaching deep into the tissues.

Particularly heartrending are the cries of addicted babies who, because of the mother's drug abuse, must detoxify right after birth. Jane, another Healing Touch practitioner, has found that short periods of smoothing or unruffling repeated every hour yield the best results. In the children's hospital of a southwestern community, Jane is a bit of a legend because her touch, often just in the energy field, brings rapid change in cranky and irritable babies.

Geriatric Care

Another largely underserved population are the elderly. For simple aches and pains to severe confusion due to organic brain changes, Healing Touch can add a valuable resource. Many psychiatric units harbor large geriatric populations that often frustrate the caregivers. We have seen a dramatic impact when nurses center together at the beginning of a shift, unruffle and transfer energy to each other as needed, and design treatment plans that include Healing Touch. Although the calming of an agitated geriatric patient may only be temporary due to neurological damage, it may be sufficient to accomplish a task or to establish rapport. A number of day treatment centers for the elderly are including Therapeutic Touch in their programs with good results, such as calming and a sense of personal empowerment. Some of the more responsive clients enjoy doing Healing Touch techniques with the other participants in the program.

Dealing with Long-Term Pain

Although the effects of Therapeutic Touch for postoperative pain have been well documented (Krieger, 1993, p. 162), less is known about the impact of energetic interventions on chronic, long-term pain. Sufferers of severe pain syndrome often travel from physician to physician looking for relief. As ever-increasing doses of pain-relieving medication are prescribed, they are prone to addiction because tolerance sets in when neurotransmitters and receptor sites become blocked. The body's capacity to produce its endorphins and enkephalins for pain relief is diminished as increasing doses of medication clog the system. All too frequently, the depression that results from years of this cycle leads to psychiatric disorder and admission to either a psychiatric care facility or a pain management unit.

Nothing moves quickly once the pattern of pain has been established, usually over several years, yet most persons in pain want instant relief, miracles on the double. It is important, then, to educate the pain patient that relief can at best be measured in increments. We may talk about a 5% improvement or a shift from level 9 discomfort to level 7. The important thing to note is that there is some shift with the energy therapy and to suggest that, from then on, gradual changes may develop over weeks and months. If there is no response whatever to the Healing Touch techniques, it is wise to conclude that the client's energy field is not able to respond energetically and that some other modality may be more appropriate.

It goes without saying that anyone with a severe pain problem should work closely under a physician's supervision. Our experience is that most specialists in this type of medicine are only too glad to have some other means of helping as they are quickly exhausted by the client's ongoing demands for medication and comforting. Thus, a number of Healing Touch practitioners are working successfully in conjunction with pain management clinics.

Patti's Story

Patti is a nurse in a hospital that combines pain management with psychiatric care. She found that pain patients disliked the unit because they felt they had different issues. Consequently, the pain patients would not participate in the community activities on the unit, and their participation in therapy groups was lackluster at best. Clearly, something else was needed. So Patti quietly began unruffling the painful areas with the clients that were open to the idea. She later taught them self-help techniques as well as relaxation skills. Participation at the evening meetings to relax before bedtime reached an all-time high when the pain patients, as well as the psychiatric patients, found they could sleep better after Patti's sessions than with medication. The patients were also more receptive and available for psychotherapy the next morning.

The patients began telling their physicians about their experiences. It took a while for the physicians to ask questions, and, when they understood what Patti was doing, they wrote a standing order for Healing Touch to be used prn (as needed), at the nurse's discretion.

SUMMARY

We can certainly say that Healing Touch has high relevance as an adjunct to medical care. There are probably as many applications of this work as the individual practitioner's interest and creativity allow. The work can be integrated unobtrusively in most health care settings and is often initiated by the consumer's request.

When approaching physicians, it is important to communicate clearly the research and scientific base and to be sensitive to the possibility of fear or personal threat on the part of traditional practitioners. Ultimately, it is the feedback from the client that is most valuable in showing how Healing Touch augments the function of a medical practice. Hence, good documentation of the initial assessment, interventions used, and evaluation of the client afterward is essential.

References

Achterberg, J. (1985). *Imagery and healing*. Boston: New Science Library, Shambala.

Chopra, D., MD (1990). *Quantum healing*. New York: Bantam Books.

Chopra, D., MD (1991). *Return of the rishi*. Boston: Houghton-Mifflin Co.

Coleman, D., & Gurin, J. (1993). *Mindbody medicine*. Yonkers, NY: Consumer Reports Books.

Dossey, L., MD (1982). *Space, time, and medicine*. Boston: Shambala Press.

Dossey, L., MD (1989). *Recovering the soul* (p. 7). New York: Bantam Books.

Gerber, R., MD (1988). *Vibrational medicine*. Santa Fe, NM: Bear and Co.

Hammerschlag, C., MD (1989). *The dancing healers*. San Francisco: HarperCollins Publishers.

Krieger, D. (1993). *Accepting your power to heal*. Santa Fe, NM: Bear and Co.

Pert, C. (1986). The wisdom of the receptors: Neuropeptides, the emotions, and bodymind. *Advances, III:3*.

13 INTERFACES WITH BODY-ORIENTED THERAPIES

Energy is the real substance behind the appearance of matter and form.

R. Stone quoted in Chitty & Muller, 1990

INTRODUCTION

This quote from the founder of Polarity Therapy reminds us of the many ways that energy-based concepts are currently being applied in body-oriented therapies. In fact, one of the most asked questions in our Healing Touch classes is how Healing Touch is related to or different from a body-oriented therapy such as massage, Reiki, or polarity.

In this chapter we will explore some of the ways that Healing Touch can be utilized readily by the body worker. The work can be integrated into the body worker's specialty practice because of its broad and basic approach to the human energy field. At the same time, it is useful to identify the ways in which Healing Touch differs from the numerous body-related therapies. Significantly, the practice of Healing Touch requires less specific anatomical knowledge and includes awareness of all the dimensions of the energy field.

BODY-RELATED THERAPIES

In the past 20 years especially, there has been increasing awareness of the physical body and ways to maintain optimum functioning. The general public began asking questions about illness, rising health care costs, and means of preventing further physical problems. Since medical science has largely focused on the diagnosis and treatment of disease, many individuals began turning to alternatives for health maintenance and self-improvement even without the consultation or approval of their physicians (Eisenberg et al., 1993). Those who chose other means of staying well began exploring the wide and growing field of body-related therapies. Many of these alternative approaches define health as a function of subtle energy that flows within the body and is obstructed or congested in illness. Thus, increasing self-awareness among the public has fostered insight about energy and intuition. Beyond physical exercise, the more adventurous seekers learned postures for stress reduction (O'Hara, 1990) and movement for relaxation and received various forms of touch therapies to soothe the body.

Body-related therapies, then, are often the layperson's first exposure to a more integrated view of the bodymind and the idea of doing more to maintain health than merely consulting one's physician. Massage, for example, has renewed its time-honored place as the art and science of muscle relaxation through specific, skillful manipulation of muscle tissue (Lidell, 1984). To assure a professional status for massage, most states require a specified number of educational hours and identified skills to license the practitioner to administer touch. Advanced training for massage therapists has led to development and certification of a wide variety of related specialty techniques — reflexology, polarity therapy, Shiatzu, and Feldenkrais, to name a few.

HEALING TOUCH AS A COMPLEMENT TO OTHER THERAPIES

Massage

Healing Touch is an excellent complement to massage therapy, especially when pain or open sores make usual deep tissue work inappropriate. It is also useful as an opening in a massage session to help prepare the client and establish rapport with the client's energy field. Another option is to use Healing Touch techniques at the end of a massage treatment to bring the other layers of the energy field into balance.

June, a licensed massage therapist, found that Healing Touch interventions allowed her to work at much deeper levels with her clients. She discovered, for example, that dense muscle tissue often separates more easily when the client is in the relaxed state that is available quickly through Healing Touch. June's clients often responded more quickly to the work in the energy field. June likens her blending of the two approaches to an etheric field massage in which all layers of the field, not just the physical, are included.

Healing Touch practice does not require the specific anatomical knowledge of massage work, although it is useful for the practitioner to have this information. To differentiate from massage, Healing Touch works either with a light touch on the body or moving the hands in the energy field above the body. Also, no draping or disrobing is required for the client to receive Healing Touch as the emphasis is on working with clients wherever they are, whether in the emergency room, in a hospital bed, in a private office, or in a home setting.

There is a wealth of information to be shared as talented body workers incorporate Healing Touch into their practices. Many of the clients are highly sensitive and ready for the multi-level work because of their personal seeking for higher levels of wellness. The following stories are examples of the interchanges of skilled body workers and sensitive, attuned clients who were able to benefit fully from the added dimension of energetic interventions.

Donna's Story

A massage client we'll call Donna complained of a lifelong problem with "tired feet." No matter what the expense, no shoes ever fit or felt right to her. As June, the masseuse, began unruffling in the energy field, Donna reported increasing discomfort and tingly sensations in her feet that she had not previously experienced. As the pain increased,

June slowed her movements, moved further out into the energy field, and gently held her focus, sending caring thoughts to Donna's entire field. Suddenly, Donna experienced an emotional and physical release, almost like an auditory pop, as the field cleared spontaneously. June completed the session by gently smoothing the problem areas and making sure Donna was fully alert before leaving the office. Since that time, Donna has had no further discomfort with her shoes and experiences living fully in her body, including her feet.

Carol's Story

Carol was a fascinating client. As a psychic consultant she was able to help many people, but her own sense of imbalance in the physical body persisted. As her massage therapist, Joe, assessed her energy field, he found marked lateral imbalance. The right and left sides of her body and face even looked different, and she described herself as "not quite together." Joe dropped his usual massage routine explaining he would work to help rebalance her field. As he proceeded with the Magnetic Unruffle, Carol felt a weaving pattern across the middle of her body, almost as if the two halves were being rejoined. Since she was highly intuitive, she saw colors ranging from yellow to blue as Joe worked, and she felt gentle releasing, like feathers brushing against the skin of her neck. Since that session, she has felt "together," lost 20 pounds, and no longer seeks traditional massage. Instead, Carol goes for monthly rebalancing of her energy field as Joe continues to learn about the colors of the human energy field from his interactions with her.

Blending with Reiki

Reiki is an ancient Sanskrit tradition that is currently growing in popularity (Lidell, 1984). Like Healing Touch, it requires centering and awareness of the multidimensional energy field. Unlike Healing Touch, the process takes about an hour and consists of a series of 12 specific hand holds on the body. In contrast, Healing Touch allows much more flexibility. As noted, some of the specific interventions listed in chapter 9 can be done in 5 minutes, and allow the healer the option of returning at a later time to do more. There is also movement with Healing Touch that permits the healer to find a problem site and to work over the most congested areas then later complete the work with transfer of energy or hand holds. So, again, the combination of the two modalities allows for optimum results through a skilled practitioner.

Integration with Deep Tissue Work

A number of body-related therapies work deep in the tissues or cause actual movement of bone. Among these we can list neuromuscular and trigger point therapies as well as craniosacral manipulation (Gordon, 1984). As we might expect, these approaches require careful training in anatomy and affect primarily the physical aspect of the energy field. The possibility of harm is a concern as each person's body may respond differently to external pressure and manipulation. In contrast, Healing Touch does not require any pressure or manipulation because trust is placed in the inner wisdom of the body and the field to respond to the gentle energy interventions in whatever way is needed.

In energy-based therapy we learn that muscles can relax one by one, sometimes over several sessions. As muscles lengthen and tension is released, bone sutures and small joints naturally realign themselves, often reversing the sequence of the injury pathway. In addition, the client has an opportunity to learn to listen to the body and note how each movement augments or diminishes relaxation.

Communication with Polarity Therapists

Polarity therapy is another form of body therapy that is currently popular. Many of the concepts taught in polarity closely resemble Healing Touch and sometimes confuse the practitioner who attempts to do both. For example, sensing energy flows with the hands is carefully taught in polarity therapy but with emphasis on direction of flows, from the negative charge to the positive, the right hand to the left hand, and so forth (Sills, 1989). Healing Touch is much more spontaneous and intuitive, emphasizing the practitioner's response to the client's unbalanced energy flows. Persons who enjoy complex cognitive learning find polarity therapy enjoyable, and the two disciplines have much to offer each other in dialogue and mutual understanding. Underlying both practices is the vision that health is a function of subtle energy flows that can be brought into balance effortlessly.

Jackie's Story

To demonstrate how complex treatment of the multidimensional human being can be, we offer the case example of a 30-year-old nurse we'll call Jackie. She attended a Healing Touch class 2 years ago, perhaps sensing that she would need more help. Her job in the intensive care unit of a midwestern hospital was highly stressful. Two weeks after taking the class, she woke up literally unable to move or to go to work. She refused medical help and had a friend bring her to a local nurse healer. The noninvasive nature of Healing Touch relaxed her enough that she could walk with care to one of the neurologists the practitioner recommended. X rays showed a herniated neck disc that would require 3 months of bed rest and close observation but no surgery, according to several medical specialists. Healing Touch then became Jackie's weekly link to a whole new world of learning about her body and her emotions.

Progress seemed terribly slow to this young woman who had been used to making quick decisions and getting things done. Her compulsive nature expressed itself in housecleaning that would strain the body and send her into acute muscle spasms. This pattern repeated itself many times until depression set in. Jackie realized that a change in lifestyle had to come from within, but she continued to struggle with doing things in her old, set ways. The Healing Touch practitioner now became a patient advocate: a link to a suitable psychiatrist to deal with the depression, a contact with the mental health counselor so that the energy field sessions could support the psychotherapy, the connector to the social worker who handled the workers' compensation aspect of the case, the liaison for ongoing dialogue with the neurologist, and the referral to massage therapy and Feldenkrais for facilitating muscle releases.

It took more than a year before Jackie was ready to seek a new job. However, she describes the difficult year as the most incredible learning experience of her life. The Healing Touch practitioner challenged her to integrate her learnings from psychotherapy, the body-oriented work, and the physicians. Jackie's specific problem of shoulder outlet syndrome required a sophisticated, multidisciplinary approach. Jackie now maintains body tone with moderate aerobic exercise, and successfully holds a more relaxed job as a rehabilitation nurse. Her own experiences in healing of the psyche and soma have become translated into an asset for helping others.

SUMMARY

In this and many similar case examples, we see how all dimensions of the energy field are involved when clients seek relief from their many tensions and old patterns. It is apparent how crucial the medical and body-related therapies are to enhancing daily functioning. The client benefits further when the medical or body-related therapist includes the adjunctive care of Healing Touch.

It remains now for us to explore the interface of energetic interventions in the outer dimensions of the energy field — the emotional, mental, and spiritual layers. As these domains are traditionally addressed by psychotherapists, we will explore the counseling applications of Healing Touch in the next chapter.

References

Chitty, J., & Muller, M. L. (1990). *Energy exercises* (p. 5). Murietta, CA: Murietta Foundation.

Eisenberg, D. M., Kessler, R. C., Foster, C., Norlock, F. E., Calkins, D. R., & Delbanco, T. L. (1993). Unconventional medicine in the United States. *New England Journal of Medicine, 328,* 246–252.

Gordon, R. (1984). *Your healing hands.* Berkeley, CA: Wingbow Publications.

Lidell, L. (1984). *The book of massage.* New York: Simon and Schuster.

O'Hara, V. (1990). *The fitness option.* Nevada City, CA: LaJolla Institute for Stress Management.

Sills, F. (1989). *The polarity process.* Dorset, England: Selement Books.

14

INTERRELATIONSHIPS WITH PSYCHOTHERAPY

*There have been many instances to convince me that
the body has memory and stores emotional experiences.
According to my understanding, at some point our
inner wisdom guides us to the opportunities to release
these stored memories, lest they block our energy flow
and weaken our life force.*

K. Shames, Healing Touch practitioner, personal
communication, August 1993

INTRODUCTION

The numerous possibilities for direct applications of Healing Touch
in the practice of psychotherapy will be explored in this chapter but
first, a word about referrals. As the case of Jackie (see chapter 13)
illustrated, a collaborative approach among various health care professionals can effect results that would not be possible with any single practitioner. We want to emphasize the importance of referrals
to other skilled practitioners to ensure the best possible care for the
client. Although it is imperative that the Healing Touch practitioner
refer for medical supervision, referrals to body-oriented therapists
with specialties beyond the techniques of energy-based work can
also be very timely and helpful. Similarly, suggesting a competent
psychotherapist is appropriate especially if emotional issues are

surfacing and the Healing Touch practitioner does not have the expertise or qualifications to do in-depth therapy.

In our experience, referrals from other health care practitioners to the Healing Touch practitioner for energy-based work are also occurring with increasing frequency. For instance, many psychotherapists are referring clients with emotional blocks or issues that are not available for talk therapy. Energetic assessment by a Healing Touch practitioner allows the client to identify lifelong patterns in the field. As the client accesses suppressed material, blocks in the energy flow can be released, and the client can then return to the original therapist for follow-up sessions. This kind of flexibility between health care professionals offers new options for clients and contributes significantly to resolving long-term problems more rapidly and to a greater depth than is otherwise possible.

HEALING TOUCH AND PSYCHOTHERAPY

Many qualified psychotherapists, such as addictions specialists, marriage and family counselors, psychologists, clinical nurse specialists, and clinical social workers, are coming to Healing Touch classes themselves. We want to address specific ways these counselors could utilize the concepts of Healing Touch and base our discussion on case examples they have shared. This is new material that is currently being presented to therapists at national conferences of psychological organizations like the Association of Transpersonal Psychology (1992, August) and the Association of Humanistic Psychology (1992, July). Further sharing and mutual dialoguing is ensuing with conferences in 1994 of psychotherapists using Healing Touch. It goes without saying that the following ideas are presented as a beginning exploration of the possibilities, not with the intent of being an exhaustive study or of making anyone a specialist in the new interface between psychotherapy and energy-based approaches.

The Work of Psychotherapists

Psychotherapists with the various backgrounds we have mentioned have an innate interest in early intervention. Whether they are aware of the layers of the energy field or not, they work with mental or emotional symptoms before they become concretized as physical problems. To put it another way, they deal with the outer layers of the energy field to prevent physical breakdown. This interest in the prevention of physical problems is manifest in the increasing literature about stress that is currently seen as the causative factor in 70–80% of physical disease (Rossi, 1986). A well-known scale actually measures in numbers the amount of distress a specific life event can cause and the likelihood of ensuing physical breakdown (Holmes & Rahe, 1967). Many of the issues that send people into psychotherapy — death of a loved one, marital discord, family strife, job-related pressures, anxiety, and experiencing a traumatic event — give opportunity for resolution at the intuitive, mental, and emotional levels of the field.

On the other hand, psychotherapists also deal with the emotional or mental distress that a physical illness or chemical imbalance can cause. We may think here of immune system dysfunction, such as Chronic Fatigue Syndrome, cancer, AIDS, or autoimmune disorders, as well as known chemical imbalances that cause emotional symptoms like endogenous depression and bipolar disorders. Many clients come for psychotherapy months, even years, after a medical operation that was emotionally devastating to them. To think in energetic terms, we could say the physical layer mended itself, but the emotional, mental, and/or spiritual dimensions need further healing.

HEALING TOUCH AS A COMPLEMENT TO PSYCHOTHERAPY

Whatever the reasons clients have for seeking therapy, Healing Touch approaches offer some very effective tools to complement the eclectic skills of the caring practitioner. The full-body techniques listed in chapter 8 can be remarkably effective when paced to the individual client's needs and selected with discernment by the counselor. Rapport is established easily through light touch or working in the field, and suppressed emotions can surface quickly in the deeply relaxed state. Apparently, the blocks in the energy field are a form of stored memory. As the therapist connects with the constricted area, the client's subconscious images, such as a repressed memory of childhood trauma, surface and can be released from the emotional layer of the field. At the same time, the therapist can assist in releasing energetic debris, and then smooth the energy layers of the chakra area to rebalance the field.

Numerous therapists have integrated Healing Touch into their practice resulting in a unique blend of energy-based concepts and counseling skills. The psychological problem areas and the condition of the energy field together give the therapist clues that can widen his resource base. In other words, the predominating emotional issue helps to determine the appropriate Healing Touch intervention that can serve as a starting place for multilevel psychotherapeutic work.

Comments from Psychotherapists

Carol Lee   Carol Lee, a clinical nurse specialist in private practice, writes:

> In my recent work, it has become apparent that I can save a lot of time and be much more connected to my client's process through monitoring the energy flow. Whereas I used to spend several sessions building trust in order that the person will eventually tell me what is affecting their health or state of '*dis-ease,*' I am utilizing Healing Touch, with its very quick feedback mechanism, to provide energetic assessments. In our collaboration, the referring physician and I both notice that I am much more aware of the subtle forces operating in our clients' lives.
>
> I have also incorporated Healing Touch prior to using psychotherapy. It is my experience that the client is then more relaxed, less anxious, more present. With clients who use compulsive chatter as a means to avoid feelings, I apply the Mind Clearing techniques, which leaves them much more relaxed and present. With clients who exhibit primarily psychological disturbances, I use Healing Touch whenever they demonstrate any physical symptoms. It seems to ease the discomfort and allow for enhanced emotional release. It is also very efficient in calming people down who are emotionally distraught or anxious.

Betty   A clinical social worker, Betty, states,

> I often use a blend of hands-on work with counseling. It seems that most people are suffering from touch deprivation rather than a lack of medication or technology in their lives. I have often witnessed the power of holding a hand or gently soothing an area of the body where there was an intense buildup of tension that the patient experienced as panic or pain in the body. In the psychiatric in-patient unit where I

worked I noticed that many people could relax, sleep, or have decreased pain after a staff or family member used some form of gentle touch. Now, with the Healing Touch skills I have specific knowledge about how I can ease a client's distress.

Jenna   Jenna is a licensed mental health counselor who also uses massage to expand her healing capacities. She states:

> As I blended massage with psychotherapy, I witnessed some profound results. If I would touch a certain area, the patient would begin to recount an earlier experience. This made more sense to me when I understood the chakras and their functions in the Healing Touch classes. I would simply move my hands in a chakra area, even without physically touching and with the client fully clothed, encouraging the client to breathe deeply and share feelings when he felt ready to talk, and memories would just pour out.
>
> A most memorable time was when I was working with a young woman who had a dense area of heavy energy in the middle abdomen. As I unruffled with my hands in the area, she remembered having gall bladder surgery in her teens. As I touched the area, her voice changed and she started wailing and sobbing. I continued gently moving my hands above the abdomen giving her ample time and space to express whatever she needed to get out. When the sobbing decreased, she described how her uncle had sexually abused her especially in the time before the operation. The memory of that time with all its agony and shame was imbedded in the surgical site and the related energetic vortex. Intense discussion of the long-suppressed event brought a sense of relief — catharsis, if you will — that would not have been possible without the clue of the energy blockage that I had picked up.

Ron   Ron is a clinical psychologist who specializes in working with AIDS patients. He finds the Mind Clearing especially effective in diminishing the effects of neuropathy that often accompany this long-term disease. If the client cannot tolerate touch, because of pain or open sores, he unruffles the painful area in the field and does the Etheric Unruffle, including time for transfer of energy. In addition, he teaches the patients and their significant others to do some daily form of centering and connection of the chakras to maintain an open flow in the energy field. With each client he does a careful review of the stress levels and helps them to explore ways of diminishing pressure and tension in their daily lives. These changes in life patterns often require a release of faulty thinking and expectations, a process that is facilitated by working with the related chakra area. Control issues, for instance, relate to the solar plexus center that may feel empty or constricted without the defense of being in charge. As the client learns to keep the center open and activates the energy of the heart center, the need for control can diminish and be released, and the person softens into a more accepting personality style.

Working through the Grief Process

The loss of a significant person is inevitable at some time or other in one's life. It has been said that all relationships end in either physical death or separation. It is, therefore, surprising that most people spend very little conscious effort preparing for death as a natural life event. The impact of a major loss can be lessened if the survivor is in otherwise good emotional health. However, if the loss comes at a time when there is already a deficit, it can have a devastating effect, disrupting the whole life pattern and emotional equilibrium.

Energetically, grief diminishes all of the chakras and the related fields. If there is underlying health, the field may bounce back each day with a simple technique such as the Full Body Balance or the Chakra Meditation. The client can learn to do this on a regular basis as a self-help technique (see chapter 15) to maintain energetic balance for the period of normal grieving that may last 1 to 2 years, depending on the significance of the loss. For people with more complex issues that have been triggered by the death, psychotherapy combined with balancing of the field is a good option.

Jean's Story

Jean was a client who suffered immobility and depression because her mother was dying "by inches" in a nursing home over many months. This kind of complicated loss where the body is still alive but the mind is unclear and the personality altered requires careful therapeutic support. The inevitable loss loomed like a monster before

Jean, yet she had no way of preparing herself for it. Resolution required helping Jean to center on a daily basis and to express all the emotions associated with her mother, including anger about her mother's past alcoholism. Rebalancing of the energy field throughout this painful process was assisted by the Magnetic Unruffle and the comforting touch of the Full Body Connection.

Shortly before her mother's actual transition, Jean was able to connect with her own spiritual resources that allowed her to see the mother's slow dying as a path of learning and to connect with a wider, more transpersonal view of the dying process.

Dealing with Depression

As with grief, depression literally depresses and diminishes the entire energy field. The difference is that depression is more pathological, causing physical symptoms of sleeping and eating disturbances and emotional lability with inability to have enthusiasm about life. The field responds more slowly to energetic interventions especially if the depression is of more than a few weeks' duration.

The Full Body Connection is usually helpful on a daily basis, and the Magnetic Unruffle is useful, if medication is indicated, to smooth the field and potentiate the effect of the antidepressant. Assessment of the chakras to find which one closes first after balancing the field may yield clues about the area that is most disturbed and in need of daily support.

Tom's Story

Tom, a businessman who was depressed for several months, experienced closing of the root chakra whenever he became angry. Because the anger could not be expressed safely in the competitive world of business, Tom's entire system would shut down and fill him with a vast sense of hopelessness and despair. Relief required awareness of the anger mechanism, finding safe outlets for his rage, and helping him to feel his body and enjoy life more fully. Initially, he did these things "just to get even" with his adversaries, but his actions put the blocked energy of the anger to work in a more constructive fashion that later gave him a sense of joy and vitality.

Managing Bipolar Disorders

The bipolar disorders in which the patient cycles between elation and depression, or manic-depressive style, appear to have their source in chemical imbalance of the body. Response to medication, again, can be enhanced with systemic applications of Healing Touch that the client can learn as self-help techniques. The major impact of energetic work as a complement to treatment is the sense of self-control the client gains. Even the worst mood swing is not so overwhelming if the client knows how to unruffle his energy field, hold the chakras, and gently comfort the body.

Overcoming Stress Reactions, Anxiety, and Phobias

Whereas depression affects approximately 20% of the population and bipolar disorders 1–2%, nearly everyone experiences stress reactions and anxiety (DSM III-R, 1987). This huge area of need can be treated with medication, but the power to overcome the obstacle has to be activated within the client. As the person explores other ways of responding to difficult life situations, she may formulate new thinking patterns, sense the peacefulness of her spiritual base, and explore ways to release negative emotions quickly.

Kimberly's Story

Kimberly worked in an office where the path to the rest room was directly in the line of sight of her supervisor. Every time she went to the rest room, she felt his piercing eyes evaluating her for wasting time. Her anxiety accelerated until she could not even imagine going to work without fear and trembling. Rather than lose her job, she decided to go to psychotherapy and resolve the conflict. In conjunction with desensitization, the therapist taught Kimberly imagery that would calm her, an affirmation or positive thought to repeat as needed, and to place her hands over the specific chakra areas of the body that felt most unprotected. Kimberly also learned how to smooth her energy field with the self-help techniques whenever she became anxious or fearful. She now is able to joke about imagining the boss's judgments of her rest room trips, helps her friends to stay centered in the office, and practices her own centering frequently.

Hyperactivity in Children

An area of growing concern in the treatment field is the care of hyperactive children. Medication is often seen as the only or most expedient approach when, in fact, children respond very well to self-management techniques. Teaching a child to meditate or center is relatively easy provided that there is some skill in pacing to the child's interests. Examples from the popular literature like the *Karate Kid* or the imagery used by Olympic athletes can build a bridge for the child to value self-mastery. Beyond that, the Healing Touch approaches of unruffling, Chakra Spread, and Mind Clearing give youngsters the opportunity to experience a calmer state of consciousness. Parents can easily reinforce the learning by offering these Healing Touch approaches on a daily basis. If nothing else, both the parents and child can gain a sense of power by dealing with their ongoing problems in a regular, caring, and systematic way. Of course, Healing Touch can easily be integrated into treatment plans that include medication and psychotherapy for hyperactivity.

Assisting with Addictions Recovery

An addiction can be defined as an emotionally backed demand for anything. This definition goes beyond the many forms of chemical dependency to include the hundreds of ways each of us may try to control others or obsess about what we think we want. These behavioral addictions are pervasive in every age group and cause untold social and personal distress. Highly addictive persons will often have major blockages in the second or third chakra areas. The depletion of energy in these major centers requires the individual to constantly seek ways of filling the void, even with substances or actions that are toxic or worsen the problem.

The key with an addictive personality is to help the individual find some way of taking personal control of the energetic imbalance. The various 12-step programs give specific guidelines for self-help and day-by-day support through meetings within a spiritually oriented framework (Sparks, 1993). Similarly, the person needs day-by-day, sometimes hour-by-hour, rebalancing of the energy field and reminders to connect with her Higher Power.

Touch, especially to smooth the field, is a quick and certain way of reconnecting with one's inner resources. In hospital settings, we have seen gentle, intentional touching calm the most frantic addictive cravings. A specific technique like Mind Clearing or the Chakra Spread can ease physical discomfort until the client can muster her inner resources and move beyond the critical moment. The self-help techniques described in chapter 15 give further resources for self-empowerment.

IMPLICATIONS FOR FAMILY THERAPY

Since Healing Touch creates a close emotional connection between practitioner and client, it is a natural device for helping families to bond. Work with couples can be enhanced by teaching them to share in sensing each other's energy fields, unruffling areas of pain, and exchanging a sequence like the Mind Clearing or the Full Body Connection. We recently worked with a couple in which the husband could not please his wife in any way. When he learned how to ease her migraine headaches using the Healing Touch approach — by unruffling the pain ridge — a whole new chapter opened in their relationship.

Working with energetic understanding allows families to welcome unborn babies as they sense the presence of the newcomer's energy field before birth. Once the infant has arrived the parents and older siblings have wonderful resources to calm baby fussiness with unruffling, transfer of energy to a specific site, and the Chakra Spread. As families grow older and their lives become more complex, the need for centering increases. Connection with the breath, setting the intent to hear each other, and working out problems with sensitivity to each person's energy field can do wonders for families in conflict.

Families constitute the largest interconnected energy field that most of us experience on a daily basis. Family therapists (Taub-Bynum, 1984) have begun exploring the family network of feelings, images, and energy as a powerful system called the Family Unconscious. With our specific understanding of the interactions between energy fields, the therapist can now work intentionally to balance the field of the entire family.

SUMMARY

Obviously, these are just indications for ways therapists might choose to work to enhance their practice. The energy-based concepts allow the counselor to comprehend the profound mystery that takes place in the therapeutic exchange. There seems to be a transfer of energy from the more centered intent of the helper to the less organized or depleted energy field of the client. We might say that the client's field begins to resonate to the higher harmony of the therapist's more intentional field. This transfer of energy is multidimensional — encompassing the emotional, mental, intuitive — and occurs mostly outside of conscious awareness. The more the psychotherapist brings energy field interaction into his awareness, the more he can monitor his own field and note subtle energetic changes in the client.

References

American Psychiatric Association (1987). *Diagnostic and statistical manual of mental disorders*, (DSM III-R). Washington, DC: A.P.A. Press.

Holmes, T., & Rahe, R. (1967). The social readjusment rating scale. *Journal of Psychosomatic Research, XI*, 213–218.

Rossi, E. L. (1986). *The psychobiology of mind body healing*. New York: W. W. Norton Co.

Sparks, T. (1993). *The wide open door*. Center City, MN: Hazelden Educational Materials.

Taub-Bynum, E. B. (1984). *The family unconscious*. Wheaton, IL: The Theosophical Publishing House.

5 SELF-CARE OF THE HEALER

A vital part of all caregiving is the clarity of the healer. In this part we will explore how Healing Touch interventions can be used for your self-care and how you can begin dialogue with the subconscious parts of yourself to increase self-knowledge. It is axiomatic that the more we know and understand ourselves the more we can be genuinely available to know and understand others.

HEALING TOUCH
FOR CARE OF THE
CAREGIVER

*Good thoughts don't make a heaven, any more than
they make a garden. . . . We are to learn first what
is heaven, and secondly, how to make it. We are to
ascertain what is right and then how to perform it.*

Florence Nightingale in Calabria & Macrae, 1994

INTRODUCTION

There is a wide discrepancy between the talk about self-care and
actual research or hands-on practice in support of this concept.
For instance, all nursing curricula teach the nurse to be a caregiver, but few single courses in our current curricula address the
needs of the caregiver. Attention to self-care is even less evident
when nurses begin their professional careers and need supportive mentoring.

THE NEED FOR SELF-CARING

My colleague and I were recently asked to present a program at the
hundred-year anniversary conference of the National League for
Nursing. Based on her research (Mabbett, 1989), we had developed
a seminar on the qualities that allow caregivers to maintain high

vitality in the workplace. Our emphasis was different from the prevailing focus on burnout in the health care field. We wanted to teach about the qualities that allow persons with high ideals to maintain their vision without succumbing to stress, apathy, and organizational pressures. As we explored these issues with the top nursing educators in the country, we asked the participants to name three items in nursing about which they were passionate. Twenty-one of the 40 respondents emphasized nursing's ability to care about others as being most significant, and 23 stated the importance of self-care for the nurse. In a different survey, 24 practitioners of nursing rated the need for self-care information to be even more important than knowledge about giving assistance to others. Self-caring, it seems, is highly desired but few know just where to begin.

Several publications are currently addressing the issues of care for the practitioner. Caryn Summers (1992) writes about the high-risk environments in which most nurses work. She estimates that more than 80% of nurses are suffering from codependency; that is, they are overly concerned with pleasing and helping others often to their own detriment. For example, chemical addiction rates are 30 times greater than for the general population, but only 13 states currently have diversion programs to address chemical dependency within the profession (Summers, 1992, p. 105). Similar statistics about nurses' vulnerability and low self-esteem were described by two nurses who summed up the dilemma in the title of their book on codependency, *I'm Dying to Take Care of You* (Snow & Willard, 1989). In addition, institutions such as hospitals seem to generate addictive patterns, causing many health care professionals to get bogged down in the mire of bureaucracy and impossible expectations (Schaef & Fassel, 1988).

Another nurse writes about her own experiences of being a "wounded healer" and the long journey to recovery in *Caring for the Caregiver* (Jarrett, 1993). Her extensive annotated bibliographies lead the reader to a variety of self-helping activities, such as exercise, nutrition, releasing dysfunctional relationships, and moving to positive inner dialogue through affirmations. The fact that publications like these are currently popular indicates that the profession is increasingly ready to face some of its own medicine and to apply a concept we have long heard: "Healer, heal thyself."

HEALING TOUCH FOR SELF-HEALING

The question is, then, who cares for the caregiver? Obviously, it must be ourselves as we look at the tremendous challenges and risks we handle on a daily basis. In our Healing Touch classes we have found that the techniques offer significant tools and starting points for self-awareness and self-nurturing. The hands-on approach of Healing Touch offers practical, powerful methods that go beyond mental control or imagery. Self-healing is the basis for transferring the focused, intentional energy that is needed to do Healing Touch with others. In the succeeding exercises we will explore self-healing work. Follow along and develop your own approaches to begin a program of genuine care of the caregiver.

Heart Centering

Each caregiving intervention begins with centering. This requires you to move within yourself to find an inner reference point or core. In contacting this inner core, you begin to find stillness and peacefulness and a sense of being unified, integrated, and focused. Centering also implies being totally present in the immediate moment and developing the ability to refocus any time the mind becomes distracted. Naturally, this requires regular practice, preferably two to three times a day for at least 15 to 20 minutes, to quiet the busy mind, relax the body, and calm the emotions. When you as a caregiver have achieved the practice of centering, you will be able to work easily in most difficult situations. As a bonus, others around you may sense your calmness and move to their own centered states of awareness more readily.

One of the most critical elements of centering is, of course, knowing when you are not in a peaceful state of mind. At first, practitioners seem to find this difficult to do because they attend mentally to the needs of the client rather than to their own internal state. Invariably, when a student of Healing Touch tells her mentors that a technique did not work, we find that centering has not been done completely enough. So we encourage potential healers to practice centering every time they feel the slightest emotional distress during the workday. The emotions are like sensors, our antennae, that allow us to receive quick feedback when something is amiss.

It is important to center from the heart chakra, the energy vortex that allows us to feel compassion and unconditional love. In using the heart-centered energy for self-healing we can also allow compassion to flow to ourselves. Heart centering can be done several times a day until it becomes an automatic response in each difficult situation. Once you become attuned to this way of self-caring, you will readily detect when you are not centered because at those times the inner voices will be judgmental and harsh. Remember, our minds and bodies have a tremendous capacity to respond to the positive suggestions we can make, especially from a centered state of consciousness.

Studies of biofeedback (Brown, 1974) show that ordinary consciousness is characterized by the beta brain wave pattern; centering shifts brain wave activity to alpha, a slower, more focused pattern. The alpha brain wave frequency allows us to increase perception and to develop our intuitive skills more readily.

EXERCISE

Heart Centering

1. Begin by allowing your awareness to move to your heart center. . . . Take a slow, deep breath and feel the energy of compassion and caring. . . . As you exhale, visualize the tension and stress in your body flowing out your hands and feet. . . . Do this three times. . . . Releasing. . . . Letting go.

2. Visualize an emerald green light at the heart center. . . . Feel the sensation of warmth and balance move into your chest . . . shoulders . . . arms . . . head . . . abdomen . . . thighs, legs, and feet. . . . Relax the entire body. . . . If the mind wanders, refocus at the heart center and repeat the process.

3. See with your inner eye a friend or someone you wish to help. Sense your heart center opening to the person in front of you and note how good it feels to send out the vibration of caring.

4. Allow the person in front of you to be yourself, perhaps as a little child or at a time that was difficult, a time you were embarrassed about something.

5. Allow that same quality of love and compassion you had for your friend to go to yourself. Forgive and feel the vibration of compassion. Allow yourself to learn from the difficult experience. Be very gentle with yourself.

6. Connect again with the breath and gently come back to full awareness.

Chakra Meditation

Many practices access a meditative state, but actually moving the hands over the chakras to activate their energies increases the effect. This meditation may be appropriate early in the morning just on awakening when the body is still at rest and the mind is starting to rustle. It is also useful to do this practice whenever you are fatigued or discouraged as it allows you to feel the vital life force flowing through the body.

EXERCISE

Chakra Meditation

1. Set your intention for the healing you wish for yourself. Begin to mobilize the healing forces within by identifying what you want to heal or release.

2. Begin with the spine in alignment, either lying down or sitting up in a comfortable position. Celebrate your aliveness with a positive statement such as, "I feel my joy; vitality is now flowing through me; I deserve love and now attract loving thoughts."

3. Releasing any tension with the out-breath, allow the hands to move to the root chakra area. . . . Feel your life force, your sense of belonging on the earth, your sense of safety and security with yourself. Hold each position for 1 to 3 minutes depending on your sense of what is needed in each area.

4. Move both hands to the sacral chakra. . . . Sense your body in balance; sense your emotional nature and ability to release what is not needed at this time.

5. Move the hands to the solar plexus area.... Notice how good it feels to protect this vulnerable area. Allow yourself to take in energy from the universe in the form of golden sunlight, wind, or ocean waves.... Sense your ability to be assertive and effective in communicating with others.

6. Move both hands to the heart center.... Feel the flow of unconditional love toward others; feel their love flowing into you. Send out the flow of this love to yourself, forgiving easily and learning from all past experiences. Feel the support of the three lower centers as you do this.

7. Move the hands to the throat center.... Sense your ability to express your being; enjoy singing, chanting, making sounds, speaking with clarity.

8. Proceed to the brow center, the intuitive chakra.... Sense your awareness expanding, able to see with insight and wisdom. See all there is to see; sense what another person's situation might be. Allow yourself an insight about a current situation.

9. Reach the crown chakra feeling your connection with the Infinite.... Unlimited resources of love and wisdom are available to you through this connection.

10. Slowly relax the hands, continuing to feel your energy flow as you move forward into the next activity of the day.

Connecting the Chakras

There are many ways of enhancing one's sense of well-being by connecting the energy centers of the major joints with the chakras related to the spinal column. One way is to follow the basic outline called "Chakra Connections" given by Brugh Joy (1979, pp. 269–274) and to personalize this exercise by adding your own variations.

The following exercise is a variation that I have found helpful. This needs to be done with a centered state of consciousness in a time frame that allows all parts of your energy system to integrate the experience. Many of our students do this practice before arising in the morning or on a break in the work schedule when they need an energy boost.

EXERCISE

Connecting the Chakras

1. Begin by acknowledging your connection with the supportive universe and sensing your inner center. Set your intention for the help you need.

2. Feeling the energy of the breath in your lungs and heart center, gently let it go to the arms and hands, then connect both hands above and below the foot on the nondominant side.

3. Move the hands higher, connecting the ankle to the knee. Hold until you feel a flow of warmth or a pulsation, a sense of aliveness, moving from the ankle to the knee.

4. Move the hands to connect the knee and hip, holding until you feel the warming flow.

5. Connect in similar fashion on the dominant side the foot, ankle and knee, knee and hip.

6. Connect both hips by letting energy flow through the hands to the hips.

7. Connect the root chakra, with one hand below or on the perineum and the other on the sacral center, just below the umbilicus.

8. When there is a flow of vitality from the feet through the lower abdomen, move higher by placing one hand on the sacral center and the other on the solar plexus. You will know exactly how much holding you need in this vulnerable area to recharge your batteries and to feel genuinely nurtured.

9. Feeling the support of all the lower centers, connect the solar plexus and heart center sensing the flow of unconditional love toward others and yourself.

10. With one hand on the heart let the other hand connect to the wrist, the elbow, the shoulder. Alternate so that the other hand is on the heart center and you connect the other wrist, elbow, and shoulder.

11. Place both hands on both shoulders giving yourself a nice big hug. Remember that all we do for ourselves is an extension of the gifts of Universal Love, of which there is a limitless supply.

12. Connect the heart chakra and the throat center, the throat and the brow, the brow and the crown. Finally, connect the crown and the transpersonal point above the crown to celebrate your connection with Higher Power as you understand it. Feel the boundaries of your marvelous energy field that extends out about as far as your hands can reach. And now you are ready for whatever is next on your agenda!

Brush Down and Shake Out

Often, we find ourselves in situations where the energy feels heavy, as when a nurse enters a hospital room full of angry family members. Remaining centered before, during, and after such an encounter requires consummate skill. Simply brushing down your own energy field to calm the jangled emotions and jagged edges of the field can be very helpful. This brushing may be a few sweeps through the entire field, head to toe, while taking some deep breaths or a smoothing of the field over the chakras that seem most vulnerable, such as the heart, solar plexus, and sacral centers.

A similar ritual is to release stagnated and sticky energy by shaking out hands and feet and moving the body in a healthy wiggle. Needless to say, these techniques may best be done away from persons who might not understand what we're doing, lest they think we have bugs or apoplexy.

Another option, of course, is to do the process mentally, visualizing your hands moving in the areas as needed. The intent is always one of providing genuine caring for self in the hundreds of difficult times that you face as a health caregiver and doing it quickly, as close in time to the triggering event as possible.

Personal First Aid

All the knowledge you have gained by learning techniques to help another person have practical applications for self-care. For instance, it is as natural to soothe a child's wound by unruffling the area over the injury as to soothe one's own wounds, burns, or cuts. The more specific technique of Ultrasound would speed healing in a concentrated area by helping a cut to mend. In more extensive injuries, such as bone fracture, repeated unruffling and Transferring Energy over the break can speed healing. Many students report good success with applying Healing Touch techniques on themselves because they can repeat the treatments as often as necessary.

LIMITATIONS OF SELF-HEALING

In our discussion of self-caring methods it is important to be clear about its limitations. The self-healing concepts work best as preventative or health maintenance tools, and they seem to be effective when utilized at the first symptom of discomfort or distress. It is self-evident that centering, a basic requirement for healing work, is difficult when symptoms are acute, such as with a migraine headache. Further, it is untenable to postpone medical treatment for any ongoing symptom that is not relieved quickly by energetic means.

Let yourself see Healing Touch as an adjunct, a complement to other treatment modalities, never as a cure-all or panacea for your mental or physical ills. Physical symptoms that need medical care may be further helped by utilizing Healing Touch. For example, pain medication is potentiated by smoothing and balancing of the field.

Emotional symptoms, similarly, may release quickly with centering and some of the self-help concepts suggested previously. For example, early signs of irritability, restlessness, fatigue, or sadness may find relief with the centering and reconnecting to the Higher Resources of the transpersonal dimension. However, energy-based concepts are no substitute for treatment of ongoing or severe symptoms such as panic attacks or depression. Good psychotherapy with skill on the part of the therapist and trust on the part of the client are needed to work out long-term issues. Interestingly, we have found that self-caring techniques such as Connecting the Chakras can be very useful in alleviating the prevalent morning "blahs" while someone is being treated for depression.

SUMMARY

All healing work is ultimately self-healing work. Almost all Healing Touch techniques described in previous chapters can be used on oneself with the only difference being that the energetic contrast will be more subtle when working on oneself than when working on another person. Hopefully, all practitioners and clients will avail themselves of this tremendous resource for health maintenance and prevention.

Because of our interest in teaching self-care to others, we have a commitment as practitioners to learning from our own experience and to teaching others from this personal understanding. Most importantly, as we apply our skills of self-caring, we are showing new possibilities to our many colleagues in need.

References

Brown, B. (1974). *New mind, new body.* New York: Bantam Books.

Calabria, M., & Macrae, J. (Eds.). (1994). *Suggestions for thought by Florence Nightingale* (p. 8). Philadelphia: University of Pennsylvania Press.

Jarrett, R. M. (1993). *Caring for the caregiver.* Beaverton, OR: Happy Talk Books.

Joy, B. (1979). *Joy's way.* Los Angeles: J. P. Tarcher, Inc.

Mabbett, P. (1989). *Maintaining vitality.* Unpublished doctoral dissertation, University of Humanistic Studies, Del Mar, CA.

Schaef, A. W., & Fassel, D. (1988). *The addictive organization.* San Francisco: Harper and Row.

Snow, C., & Willard, D. (1989). *I'm dying to take care of you.* Redmond, WA: Professional Counselor Books.

Summers, C. (1992). *Caregiver, caretaker.* Mt. Shasta, CA: Commune-a-Key Publications.

16

THE PERSONAL DEVELOPMENT OF THE HEALER

People will do anything, no matter how absurd, in order to avoid facing their own souls.

Jung, 1974

If we are free in ourselves, we can free others. If we are binding people to ourselves, then we are not ourselves free, and we cannot free others.

Khan, 1982

INTRODUCTION

Our discussion of self-care of the healer makes it clear that the energy field of the healer is the resource for healing. If we are free of emotional debris, we can be a connector or facilitator for the client in helping to make available the vast potential of the Universal Energy Field. If we are blocked in some way or out of balance, we cannot assist with this connection. In other words, there are no secrets in energy-based work: in the same ways that we sense the client's field with our Higher Sense Perception, so we are perceived by the client as the transfer of subtle energies occurs.

In this chapter we will explore some of the major areas of self-development that can provide ways for you to move more deeply into your inner awareness and develop precious, internal resources.

COMMUNICATION WITH THE CLIENT

It is well known in communication theories that nonverbal signals are much more powerful than verbal ones. Our understanding of energy fields in human interactions supports this idea. Think, for instance, of the many times we express feelings of closeness or intimacy with another as "good vibrations" or "being in harmony." From an energetic point of view this is very accurate — some level of the healer's being, perhaps one that is barely in conscious awareness, reaches the client and seems to lift his depleted vibrations to a higher level.

One of the silver rules of psychotherapy is that the client can go no further than the therapist has dared to venture in her own explorations of the complex forces of the subconscious mind. By the same token, an unaware caregiver can be drawn into the client's more constricted field and become quite depleted. It is not so much that the client is generating some form of negative energy, as energy is basically neutral, but that the diminished field can establish a resonance of its own and similar areas of tension in the healer also become activated. So we can understand energetically the old therapeutic maxim that either the client gets better or the therapist gets worse.

Working with subtle energies means careful pacing to the client's needs so that we do not overwhelm by bringing in too much energy or are not overly sympathetic, which renders us incapable of lifting to a higher level to help the client. This ability to be as aware as possible and to pace correctly in language and energetic flow requires an exquisite commitment to one's own learning.

PERSONAL DEVELOPMENT TECHNIQUES

The essential qualities of the healer, then, are a dedication to personal development, a commitment to keep gaining from our experiences, an openness to new ideas, enthusiasm to take on the great adventure of life, and a willingness to work through personal difficulties with an attitude of flexibility.

Jung (1974), the great teacher of inner knowing, said that the first part of our life is spent finding our personal identity, and the second part of life is moving into our greater identity as spiritual and mature beings. He called this maturing *individuation* to differentiate from the achievement-oriented nature of our early life's work. Anyone who is serious about healing needs to individuate — to be less dependent on others' opinions and be able to hear the inner guidance that is available through daily, committed practice.

Journal Writing

One of the most effective ways to start the inner dialogue with the many layers of your inner being is by journal writing (journaling). A number of fine resource books are available to describe specific approaches (Cappachione, 1991; Progoff, 1975; Rainer, 1978), but the most important thing is to get started. It is helpful to have an attractive notebook that is available to you any time you wish to write and that is completely private. You might want to think of journal writing as writing letters to yourself as you begin to open dialogue with unknown parts of yourself. As no new friendship could develop without regular communication, so this dialogue with the inner being, your own best friend, needs to be comfortable, enjoyable, and frequent.

The journal becomes a place for expressing feelings you may never have shared, for exploring ideas, or for reflecting on events in your life. This is not a clinical record or a log of daily activities, but rather a place to describe subjective experiences, images, gut reactions, and future goals and to celebrate an internal victory. Some people find it useful to use the journal to set the goals, the intent, and the energy for the day in the morning and then to review these items at the end of the day, noting what has been resolved and what is in need of further action. Another way to increase your communication repertoire might be to write letters, which you don't necessarily send, to friends and adversaries. The key is creative self-expression and sensing the center of your being. The journal thus becomes a place where you experience your inner "home base."

Dream Work

If journal writing provides an avenue for reaching out to the deeper self, dream work gives us windows into the inner world. To quote a great teacher, "Dream psychology opens a way to a general comparative psychology from which we may hope to gain the same understanding of the development and structure of the human psyche as comparative anatomy has given us concerning the human body" (Jung, 1974, p. 34). Although many dreams appear mysterious because of their symbolic nature, they are a self-portrait of something that is actually at work in the subconscious mind. Even a brief fragment or an emotion that we remember can give us some idea of the inner psyche and the unfolding self.

Some easy ways to track dreams and learn from the inner teacher are to set your intent to learn from a dream memory and have a pad, pen, and flashlight on hand when going to sleep. On awakening, write down the image, symbol, or emotional fragment before doing anything else, as activity disrupts the memory patterns. Even if you get only a small fragment, thank your inner being for the information. Remember that you are building a relationship with the unknown, deeper parts of yourself.

As you progress in getting more dream material, you may wish to sort out themes and patterns. This has to be done with the utmost respect since we know that any external friend would be frightened by criticism or judgment. Many books (Johnson, 1986; Thurston, 1978) give excellent tools for self-understanding.

EXERCISE

Dream Work

1. Begin by writing down as many key words associated with the dream as possible. Look at the key words you have written down and quickly make as many associations with each word as possible. For example, "woman" may be associated with mother, feminine, soft, comfort, old, wise, etc.

2. As you review the overall quality of the dream, certain associations will fit more precisely than others. There will

be a sense of recognition. Note the associations that fit for the dream.

3. Begin to notice how the key words fit into a pattern, an overall observation or general statement that can be made, such as "The dreamer is always in some kind of trouble."

4. Allow yourself to think of ways this might be true for you and what message you can specifically draw from the statement.

5. Allow some action to follow, either writing down your insights, celebrating your awareness in some way, or doing something specific and practical.

A colleague reported that she utilized this way of working with dreams. "In the early explorations of my own inner world," she states, "I had several repeated dreams about my car being out of control and some kind of fire in the rear end of it. I tried to look for associations with control issues but found no resolution that fit. After the dream kept repeating, I moved to action and took the car to a garage for a long overdue checkup and found that the brake linings, especially in the rear, were almost totally burned out."

It is interesting to note that many of our students report dreams of doing or learning Healing Touch. The healing archetype, as it is exemplified in Healing Touch, is very much alive and needed in our troubled world. One dreamer described in detail learning how to do the Chakra Spread technique before it was presented in the classroom. Another student spoke of many regrets about not being at her mother's bedside at the time of the mother's transition. In a dream she was able to do the Magnetic Unruffle with her mother, and floods of tears as she told the story affirmed the validity of inner healing. In a different vein, a very young participant dreamed the whole earth was on fire with pollution and chaos. In her despair, she began to smooth out the earth's energy field and to get some relief from the tension.

Activating the Three Injunctions

As mentioned, all inner explorative work must be done with care and respect. Brugh Joy (1979, pp. 60–61) tells the story of a very intuitive woman who was seeking self-understanding and heard a voice giving three specific instructions for her development. The three instructions appear as basic rules for operating in the self-exploratory, intrapersonal dimension: (1) Make no comparisons. (2) Make no judgments. (3) Delete your need to understand.

In a culture where achievement is highly valued, comparisons seem essential, and we are constantly trying to meet our own or others' high expectations. Judgments keep us locked in a prison of predictable patterns with little opportunity for new ideas or opening to others. The need to understand locks us into patterns of trying to analyze and figure out everything with little room for accepting and enjoying the mystery of life.

Therefore, comparisons, judgments, and overanalysis can be the basis of a workaholic lifestyle and an obsessive-compulsive personality pattern, or they can drive us to stress-related disease and premature death by heart attack or fatigue. To counteract these trends, working with the three injunctions gives us a chance to break out of these barriers. The following exercises can be used to break unwanted thinking patterns until new ones become natural and automatic.

EXERCISE

To Decrease Comparisons

1. Ask your inner self to help you to be aware each time you make a comparison. The comparisons may be between yourself and others (Joe is smarter/dumber than I am) or between other people (Mary's car is better/worse than Alice's car).

2. At the end of the day, write down the approximate number of these comparisons.

3. After a while, you may wish to set your intent to change these unnecessary thought patterns. Then you can catch yourself midsentence or midthought and reprogram the thought.

4. Work throughout the day with your intent to be less evaluating and to become more accepting simply of things as they present themselves.

EXERCISE

To Diminish Judgments and Criticism

1. Starting with your awareness of judgmental thoughts, move to cancel or erase the thoughts and words you really don't mean.

2. Notice that most people are quite understanding when you go through a process of increasing self-awareness such as this. In fact, they may be encouraged to try being less judgmental themselves because of your efforts.

3. As often as possible note how something you have done is interesting, rather than going to negative self-statements such as, "Boy, was I dumb."

4. Remember to let your higher self observe the ego's antics with humor and a quality of being a "fair witness." So instead of berating yourself, you might share an observation like, "Mary disagreed with me and I was hurt and started to withdraw. How interesting."

Deleting the need to understand means to drop *your* need to analyze things that are beyond comprehension. It certainly does not mean leaving your inquisitive nature or knowledge base behind. As we move in the path of learning about the deeper self, we often experience a coming together of unusual events, *synchronicities* as Jung called them, that suggest we are being led to new learning. For instance, many students report finding information about an upcoming class just when they received an unexpected check in the mail. Trying to figure out events like these could slow down the flow of life and take away the fun of enjoying the mysterious. In extremes, we see persons with "paralysis of analysis," unable to move with spontaneity because everything has to be understood or planned on the mental level. In working to diminish your need for constant mental comprehension, you may want to journalize at the end of each day. Note unusual events and trends that seem to be unfolding.

Creative Self-Expression

Another way to connect with one's inner resources is through creative self-expression. Since our goal is learning about the subconscious levels within, no artistic skill is needed here. Rather, use whatever medium is most suitable to express parts of yourself that might otherwise remain hidden. The secret, as always, is in centering first and remaining free of all judgmental or limiting thoughts.

Mandala Drawing   Mandala drawing is an age-old technique in which one works with a circle on paper and allows the circle to fill either from the inside to the outer edges or from the outer rim to the middle. This is an example of a simple focusing device; you can use crayon, colored pencils, or pastels. As your interest progresses, you may enjoy the research that has been done utilizing mandala drawing as a form of art therapy (Kellogg, 1977) or Jung's perception of the mandala as a cross-cultural phenomenon of spiritual expression (Jung, 1972).

Object Arrangement   Another easy way to connect with the inner being is through object arrangement. We often spontaneously gather up objects that have special meaning to us and create a place in the home for this collection. Doing this intentionally with the idea of making a meditation space could be one way of connecting safely with the deep. This way of focusing can become highly therapeutic when, for instance, we assemble all the symbols evoking the memory of a friend to celebrate an event or to assist with grief work (Kazanis & Hover-Kramer, 1990).

Creative Play   Whatever the medium or the structure, let this be a time of flowing with your tools, feeling the movement of the inner rhythm and appreciating the results, however crude they may be. Jung regularly allowed an hour a day for sand play in his busy schedule, building cities, castles, and mandalas to have private, personal communication time that gave him immense satisfaction. Since then, whole schools of sand play techniques have evolved to utilize this delightful medium. Singing, dancing, or simply moving to music are other ways of playing without any particular intent other than self-discovery. The goal in creative play is to learn to trust the inner knowing and to recapture the spontaneity and joy that we knew as children.

Meeting the Shadow

Self-knowledge means facing all parts of ourselves, even the parts we do not like. The shadow side of the personality is the designated bearer of the unknown and can be highly destructive if we ignore it. Notice, for example, how much easier it is to blame or shift feelings to someone else than to actually own the unpleasant parts of ourselves. Our conscious mental mechanisms are actually designed to suppress what is unpleasant and, often, most important. Just as we have a blind spot when driving that causes accidents unless we learn to compensate, so we must learn to track this shadowy side of ourselves and learn its lessons.

A helpful way to begin tracking the shadow is to note the persons we dislike in an irrational way. Ask yourself what quality is most despicable about this person and how this might relate to something within you. For example, a healer found himself despising a certain client who was dependent and whiny. Instead of judging or withdrawing from the client, he asked what he could learn from the situation. In looking hard at his own hidden dependency needs, the healer was able to reconcile opposites within himself and see the client with more compassion.

Projection   When the shadow side is not confronted, we are likely to project our own uncomfortable feelings onto another. In the healing process, this countertransference, as it is known in the psychological literature, is a severe limitation to the therapeutic alliance. Energetically, the flow of unlimited potential from the universal through the healer is blocked. We may label a client as "difficult" or "unresponsive" when, in fact, *we* may be the persons who are unresponsive to significant client clues because of our own blind spots.

Worse, of course, is the projection of our unwanted parts onto a whole group of people. History abounds with examples. The Puritans of New England, for instance, liked things to be nice and tidy. "They feared swarthy Indians, probably were suspicious of dark-feathered turkeys, and walked uneasily in the pitchy pine woods of Massachusetts. For women they advised stockings, hoods, obedience, and silence. Hatred of the Yin side of the circle begins as a small thread in the first American cloth. Hatred of Yin at the start gave New England a fierce energy; but three hundred years later, the same hatred drains people and leads to some sort of spiritual death" (Bly, 1988, p. 11).

These words recapture for us the power of the unconscious forces to evoke fear and projection when they are not understood. Thousands of healers, mostly women, who attuned to the mysteries of nature at a time when their cultures were overly rational, were burned as witches in the not too distant past.

As we learn about the personal shadow, we can also understand these mass projections. Although there may be no formal witch hunts, there are hundreds of ways that the intuitive can be discounted and flattened. Since the reconciliation of our internal opposites is primary, we always begin by addressing the personal issues. From this daily work of self-awareness can come an attitude of inner harmony and peacefulness that allows us to face more public discounts or distractions with relative ease and non-defensiveness, without projection hooks for others to latch onto. Reclaiming the shadow and integrating it allows us to acknowledge the unpleasant parts of ourselves but also to let the giant within emerge (Bly, 1988, p. 42).

OPENING TO THE TRANSPERSONAL PERSPECTIVE

The word *transpersonal* refers to the dimension of human consciousness that is greater than the personal, a *meta-* or *super*personal awareness. This connection with the dimension greater than the individual self is part of the spiritual journey that begins as we ask deeply about the meaning of life and death. This questing is quite distinct from a religious perspective that encompasses a set of specific beliefs and social forms of expression. Instead, the transpersonal refers to a worldview, an attitude, a process of self-discovery, and an expansion beyond the merely personal (Small, 1991).

Many therapists and counselors are exploring spiritual dimensions as they look toward helping the sickness of the soul. The Association of Transpersonal Psychology is a focal point of the increasing dialogue between therapists and spiritually oriented teachers, and it seems evident that the work of Healing Touch belongs in this context since it addresses the multidimensional nature of humans.

Use with Self-Healing Techniques

The perspective that allows us to see ourselves as spiritual beings having human experiences lifts and transforms our dilemmas and permits a wider dimension of self-healing to take place (Hover-Kramer, 1989). In her study of 35 caregivers, a nursing researcher found that working with the transpersonal, and allowing oneself to see a bigger picture, created a sense of meaning in difficult situations. Burnout among caregivers was significantly reduced when they moved beyond feelings of loss and devastation by evoking their connections with the Higher Self and a sense of meaning. "What emerged from the interviews as an over-riding theme of caring was the experience of spiritual transcendence. Spiritual transcendence was defined as experiencing oneself in relationship as a part of a force greater than oneself. This spiritual transcendence experience was critical not only in terms of the nurses' satisfaction with caring, but also as an explanation of the paradox of distance and closeness . . ." (Montgomery, 1991, p. 36).

As the traditions of self-healing through Alcoholics Anonymous and the related 12-step programs bear out (Mikluscak-Cooper & Miller, 1991; Small, 1991), problems are never solved at the level at which they were created. With our understanding of energy, we know that we vibrate to the same frequency as that to which we give primary attention. When we are bogged down in ordinary consciousness ruminating about an issue, we are vibrating at the energetic frequency of the problem. When we allow our perspective to shift, to attend to the Universal Will for the situation, we lift our vibrational frequency, just as a musician can raise a tone by going to the higher octave. The following exercise allows you to be aware of a problem and to let it change by looking at it with a different perspective, a different level of consciousness.

EXERCISE

Moving to the Transpersonal Perspective

1. Be aware of a problem that holds tension for you at this time. Allow yourself to look at the problem through your own eyes.

2. Now, see the same problem through the eyes of someone who disagrees with you.

3. Note the impasse this creates.

4. Using your skills of centering and focused meditation, lift higher. Imagine you are looking at the whole thing from above, from an eagle's point of view, or how Higher Power as you understand it might see the issue.

5. See someone you highly respect, say Buddha or Jesus or Mary, handling the situation.

6. Bring this awareness to the present situation, applying your new insight with compassion for yourself and the others involved.

Being in touch with our spirituality is, thus, not only uplifting but may indeed be life-saving when we think of the tremendous price our culture is currently paying through stress-related illnesses and helper burnout. "Humans have a profound need for transpersonal experiences and for states in which they transcend individual identities to feel their place in the large role that is timeless" (Grof & Bennett, 1992, p. 116). Apparently, this is part of our human development: to go beyond our ego selves, to evolve, and to develop the farther reaches of our human natures.

SUMMARY

We have attempted to outline some of the ways you might begin your personal quest for inner development. There are many paths, such as journal writing, dream work, paying attention to our inner dialogue, expressing creatively, meeting the shadow, and opening to the transpersonal perspective. Your work as a healer requires full awareness of yourself so that you can genuinely attune to others. The desire to help is the beginning, then, of a lifelong journey of self-discovery and increasing intrapersonal richness. It is a quest that is ever rewarding and expanding to facilitate your connection with others.

References

Bly, R. (1988). *A little book on the human shadow*. San Francisco: Harper and Row.

Cappachione, L. (1991). *The picture of health*. Santa Monica, CA: Hay House.

Grof, S., & Bennett, H. Z. (1992). *The holotropic mind*. San Francisco: Harper and Row.

Hover-Kramer, D. (1989). Creating a context for self-healing: The transpersonal perspective. *Holistic Nursing Practice, 2:3.*

Johnson, R. (1986). *Inner work*. San Francisco: Harper and Row.

Joy, B. (1979). *Joy's way*. Los Angeles: J. P. Tarcher, Inc.

Jung, C. G. (1972). *Man and his symbols*. Princeton, NJ: Bollingen Series.

Jung, C. G. (1974). *Dreams*. Princeton, NJ: Bollingen Series.

Kazanis, B., & Hover-Kramer, D. (1990). Object arrangement. *Beginnings, 10:4.*

Kellogg, J., MacRae, M., Bonny, H., & Di Leo, F. (1977). The use of the mandala in psychiatric evaluation and treatment. *American Journal of Art Therapy, 7*, 123–134.

Khan, P. V. I. (1982). *Introducing spirituality into counseling and therapy*. Lebanon Springs, NY: Omega Press.

Mikluscak-Cooper, C., & Miller, E. (1991). *Living in hope*. Berkeley, CA: Celestial Arts.

Montgomery, C. (1991). The caregiving relationships, paradoxical and transcendent aspects. *Journal of Transpersonal Psychology, 12:3.*

Progoff, I. (1975). *At a journal workshop*. New York: Dialogue House.

Rainer, T. (1978). *The new diary*. Los Angeles: J. P. Tarcher, Inc.

Small, J. (1991). *Awakening in time*. New York: Bantam Books.

Thurston, M. (1978). *How to interpret your dreams*. Virginia Beach, VA: A.R.E. Press.

CONCLUSION WITH OPENING TO NEW QUESTIONS

At some point we need to decide whether the Great Picture that surrounds us is friendly or not.

Hover-Kramer, 1994

INTRODUCTION

As we come to the conclusion of this exploration of Healing Touch, we recognize that there are many new questions. We have attempted to give some of the historical basis of this work as part of the evolving new paradigm in health care — the emphasis on complementary and alternative approaches from a more integrative and holistic perspective. As the rubric of health care is expanding and evolving at a rapidly accelerating rate, the understandings of touch, interpersonal relationships, and the importance of the transpersonal dimension in healing are shifting. These changes may create whole new ways of looking at modalities such as Healing Touch.

PROGRESS IN THE CONCEPT OF HEALING

One very clear trend is that the word *healing* is no longer taboo in clinical settings. That the power for healing is within the client or patient is also increasingly accepted. Utilizing

Scandrett-Hibdon's model of endogenous healing allows us to recognize the full participation of the individual and his capacity for choice-making. To put this into practice will require continued effort, skill, and insight on the part of the caregiver. As a beginning, some hospitals are currently attempting to humanize their settings, to develop active programs of patient education, and to facilitate patient self-responsibility. Caregivers will need extensive training and increased awareness of human interactions and field effects. These learnings will allow the caregiver to maximize the endogenous, participatory process of healing.

Another dimension leading to new questions is the ongoing research into energetic phenomena. The newly formed California Institute of Human Science provides a setting for graduate studies as well as for research into the meridians and transpersonal psychobiological effects (Motoyama, 1994). Another example is the recent funding through the NIH Office of Alternative Medicine of 30 research projects in nontraditional models. This is the first time that national funding has been extended to complementary approaches, signifying increased recognition of the new paradigm. Unfortunately, funding is very slim as witnessed by the $30,000 awarded to Dr. Deepak Chopra to study the effects of 5,000-year-old Ayurvedic practices at his newly formed Mind Body Institute in San Diego (Sharp Health Care Foundation, 1994). We can only hope that this is indicative of increasing interest and funding into what really happens in the healing process.

It is the essential nature of the scientific perspective to take observed phenomena, study them, research them, and draw tentative conclusions that can lead to possible theories. We are attempting to do this carefully in considering the healing stories of many of our clients and the case examples of this book. As yet we do not have the objective studies and replication to confirm a specific theory of healing or its methods. We can point to the relevance of human caring, intentionality on the part of the healer, and understanding of our transpersonal natures as partial explanations. In reality, all of the studies mentioned in the research chapter are beginning explorations pointing to further questions.

One of the finest medical theorists today, Dr. Larry Dossey, posits that public awareness has shifted from the mechanical, material view of physical medicine to mindbody medicine, and beyond that, to a nonlocal and transpersonal perspective (Dossey, 1993, pp. 40–41). We are looking not only at the more complex ways the mind and emotions impact the body and its health, but at the ways in which expanded consciousness creates a bridge between persons. He sees mind as both local and nonlocal; the nonlocal dimension of our being is unbounded and infinite in space and time permitting the possibility of healing at a distance and between human energy fields.

SUMMARY

With this we may have a beginning framework for the good news: we are not alone. Those of us who genuinely wish to set intentionality for healing have resources from which to draw. Healing is a multidimensional process encompassing our full physical, emotional, mental, and spiritual faculties. As helpers we are no longer limited to wishes for physical curing, since often the complex biochemical changes of chronic or severe dysfunction are irreversible in the material plane. We still have much work to do in facilitating release, resolution, and new balance in the other dimensions.

The story of little Paul in chapter 1 did not end with his physical transition from life. Instead, there is an ongoing evolution of the emotional and spiritual life of his family and his essence in many dimensions. We just had the privilege of learning with him for a brief time.

Likewise, the story of Healing Touch does not end with this book. As we practice the techniques, we will learn new approaches from our clients. As we center ourselves, we will open to new levels of self-awareness. As we encounter difficulties, we will ask many more questions. As we observe the phenomena around us, we will develop new theories about healing. We as caregivers and healers are part of an ongoing, evolutionary process that opens to ever-new possibilities.

> At the deepest level of the individual
> Lies the Soul
> The part of yourself that touches higher consciousness
> And reaches out to the heartbeat of humanity.
> It leads you gently
> From enchantment to awakening
> From bondage to liberation
> From fear of death to immortal life
> From local time to the eternal Present.

References

Dossey, L., MD (1993). *Healing words*. San Francisco: HarperCollins Publishers.

Motoyama, H. (1994). On self-realization. *CIHS Newsletter, 1:2.*

Sharp Health Care Foundation (1994, January). National Institutes of Health fund Sharp research grant. *Mind Body Connection.*

A Intake Assessment

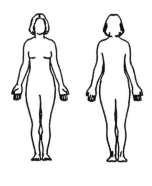

Name: _____

Address: _____

Phone #: _____

Age: _____

Occupation: _____

Living Situation:

Meditation Experience:

Health Care Professionals:

Reason for Coming:

Relevant Medical Information:

Medications:

Stress Experienced:

Relaxation:

Date: _____ Session #: _____

Appendix

B | The Certification Process to Become a Certified Healing Touch Practitioner

(Presented with permission from the Certification Board of the American Holistic Nurses' Association, © copyright 1994.)

The purpose for awarding certification as a Healing Touch Practitioner is to document the collected experiences of the individual, to acknowledge competent and experienced practice based on an established educational program, to identify and acknowledge the new professional, and to communicate with the public by recognizing this educational preparation. The certificate ensures that the participant in the program has achieved a level of skill and personal growth that is comparable to others at the same level of expertise.

The following criteria must be met for certification:

1. Completion of all coursework for the Healing Touch Practitioner: Level I, Level II-A, Level II-B, Level III-A, Level III-B.

2. Evidence of receiving ten different healing modalities with professionals; evidence of giving 100 Healing Touch sessions of which the ten best are documented in paragraph form.

3. Development of a professional profile notebook which includes a comprehensive resume, articles written by or about the individual, detailed listing of conferences and educational experiences related to professional practice.

4. A brief resume of all education, licenses, and experience, including Healing Touch workshops, dates, places, and instructors.

5. Mentorship with a certified Healing Touch practitioner for one year or more, documented by a written evaluation of the experience by the mentor and a self-report from the individual.

6. Evidence of ongoing reading and related educational experiences described in paragraph form (15–20 books, tapes studied, conferences attended, etc.).

7. A descriptive case study of work in depth with one client to demonstrate a minimum of 3–5 sessions including intake, assessment, treatment planning, implementation, evaluation, referrals, and discharge planning.

8. A self-study describing personal development throughout the educational program, plans for continued personal and spiritual growth, development of the practice of Healing Touch in the community and in the world as a whole.

I N D E X

A

Abuse, childhood, energy fields and, 87–88
Acceptance, endogenous healing process and, 20
Acupuncture, 13
Addictions recovery, 197–198
Addictive processes, sacral chakra and, 63
Adrenal glands, root chakra and, 62
AIDS
  energy field and, 80
  heart chakra and, 65
Ajna center, 66
Alignment, endogenous healing process and, 21
Allergic reactions
  energy field and, 82
  sinus headaches and, 150
American Holistic Nurses' Association, Healing Touch program and, 28, 165
Anahata, 64–65
Anxiety, 196
Appraisal, endogenous healing process and, 19–20
Arthritis
  energy field and, 82
  identifying, 142
  treatment of, magnets and, 16
  ultrasound and, 123–124
Association of Humanistic Psychology, 190
Association of Transpersonal Psychology, 190
Asthma, energy field and, 82
Astral body, 53
  described, 51
Astral light, 47
Aura, 49, 53
  described, 51

  dysfunction of, 52–53
Autoimmune diseases
  energy fields and, 82
  heart chakra and, 64–65
Awareness, endogenous healing process and, 18–19
Ayurvedic medicine, 171, 228

B

Back problems
  identifying, 142–147
  meaning of, 147
Bailey, Alice, 60
  conditions of chakras and, 72
Beck, Robert, healers' brain wave patterns and, 18
Becker, Robert, use of electricity, 16
Biofield
  acknowledged by Hippocrates, 11
  terms for, 12
Biorhythms, crown chakra and, 67
Bipolar disorders, 196
Birthing, Healing Touch and, 175–176
Blockage, release, vertebrae, 144
Blocked chakras, effect of, 78
Blue
  brow chakra and, 66
  throat chakra and, 65–66
Body, lower, connecting, 143
Body-related therapies, 182
  deep tissue work and, 185
  massage, 182
  polarity therapists and, 186
  Reiki and, 185
Bones, fractured, 147–148